The Sex
Diaries

ACKNOWLEDGEMENTS

As you've just learned, peeking behind office doors can be every bit as sexy as bedroom doors. And the offices here at Sex Diaries HQ have been bustling this year, thanks to the hard work of my agent, Todd Shuster, who has always believed in this project, and Esmond Harmsworth, who immediately knew that his home country *needed* the Sex Diaries, and made this book possible.

This book would not exist without the brilliant work of Luisa Metcalfe, who was instrumental in collecting Diaries and communicating with Diarists, not to mention the pivotal task of translating British English for me. Thank you, Luisa, for clarifying the nuances of *shag* and *arse,* as well as confirming that, no, 'cock up' does not mean what I think it does.

The anonymous Diarists, of course, deserve the bulk of the praise, for not only *writing down* their inner lives – a task in itself – but for going out on a limb and sharing them with the world. Diarists, this is the most public thank you possible, so I thank you for sharing your stories. I love my Diarists. You are amazing people with incredible stories, and made creating this book far too much fun.

Thank you to Ellen Breslau at *Woman's Day* magazine for her flexibility, and for not batting an eye when I spontaneously began handing in American columns in Anglicised English. And thank you to Long Tall Sally (longtallsally.com) for making me look every bit the confident, long-limbed editor, with a wardrobe that is every tall girl's dream.

Thank you to Betty Dodson and Diana Adams, whose sheer existence and dedication to relationship truth helped me believe that a book like this might be possible.

And lastly, I'd like to thank my ex-partners for their many positive and negative influences. This book would not have come about without them, and certainly not without the support of the love of my life, Nate Guisinger, who I am now quite certain is the best partner in the world.

WANT TO KNOW WHAT HAPPENS NEXT?

Catch up with the Diarists at TheSexDiariesProject.com, or sign up to keep your own Diary.

The Sex
Diaries

edited by Arianne Cohen

Vermilion
LONDON

1 3 5 7 9 10 8 6 4 2

This edition published 2013
First published in 2011 by Vermilion, an imprint of Ebury Publishing
Ebury Publishing is a Random House Group company
Originally published by Vermilion in 2011 as *The Sex Diaries Project*

The Random House Group Limited Reg. No. 954009

Addresses for companies within the Random House Group can be found at
www.rbooks.co.uk

A CIP catalogue record for this book is available from the British Library

The R   'ship
    Cc   n
    organ   iC®-
certified   l by the
    leading   paper
procuren   onment

ISBN 9780091939557

Copies are available at special rates for bulk orders. Contact the sales
development team on 020 7840 8487 for more information.

To buy books by your favourite authors and register for offers, visit
www.randomhouse.co.uk

This book is a work of non-fiction based on the life, experiences and recollections
of the Diarists. In some cases names of people, places, identifying characteristics
or the detail of events have been changed or obscured to protect the privacy of others.

CONTENTS

MARRIED

WHEN RELATIONSHIP BECOMES LIFESTYLE

EJECTED FROM THE RELATIONSHIP

INTRODUCTION

I have the best job in the world: I collect Sex Diaries. Dozens per week, filled with pleasure and heartache and pining and love and kink and delicious fantasies brought to life.

You probably grabbed this book because of the word 'sex' in its title. You've chosen well: the pages ahead chronicle the titillating happenings behind the bedroom (and kitchen, bathroom and closet) doors of your comely neighbours and sultry strangers, in tantalising bite-size portions. Now you get to join in as they relive Tuesday's mind-blowing sex, breath by breath, or take you along on their erotic date night.

I too began my flirtation with the Sex Diaries based on the allure of sex, when I snagged a freelance assignment for an American magazine. The idea was simple: to capture what people were really thinking about and experiencing in their bedrooms and relationships. I instructed the Diarists to include all sexual and relationship thoughts, behaviours and arousals, and to keep it brief. The article became a cover story that flew off the shelves, and then an outrageously popular online column, where readers eagerly awaited their weekly Monday afternoon peek into some-one else's sex life, hooked by the opportunity to voyeuristically look in on their neighbours' sex and relationship lives in tantalising four-minute dips. You have no idea of the chaos that erupted in my inbox if I ran late!

Yes, you will read a lot of sex in this book, in ways and strategies that will keep you captivated. But the Diaries are a phenomenon because they are not just about sex: they are about all the ways (emotionally, romantically, physically) that people just like you connect with – and disconnect from – others. Relationships are the centrepiece of our lives, and sex a prime way in which we connect, yet rarely do we see the spicy options, and have the context to compare ourselves.

This urge to know what your neighbours are up to is a natural one. Until a few thousand years ago, everyone knew everything about everyone. If your fellow hunter-gatherer could only get off with his loincloth stuffed in his mouth while screaming unsweet-nothings, you knew about it! Now we only know what we accidentally hear through the walls, which is an odd state of affairs.

The voyeurism of this book, it turns out, is an excellent use of your time. In fact, it is by witnessing others' behaviour that we gain permission to try it ourselves. This collection enables you to enter the minds behind a wide array of lifestyles and strategies. Perhaps you'll transform from a foggy sense of sexuality to a more enlightened orientation. Or be inspired by one of the numerous ways that people come together and share their souls and their bodies. If you're not happy with where you are, a flip through *The Sex Diaries* may very well give you a whole new game plan.

This book marks the international expansion of the project, with a whole tome devoted to the relationship and sexual lives of people around the British Isles, alongside sister US and Italian books, and www.sexdiariesproject.com.

I am often asked whether the Diaries are a mirror of relationships and sexuality in Great Britain. Goodness, no! This is a collection, not a statistical survey, and my aim is to create a portrait of contemporary

British sex lives, allowing readers to discover what their neighbours are really up to.

How do I know that the Diaries are real? The project began and continues as a journalistic project, with truth as its driving mission. Though I cannot personally witness the Diarists' experiences (and my doe eyes are quite content with this state of affairs), my frequent phone conversations with Diarists confirm and elaborate details, and all Diarists' circumstances are vigorously fact-checked.

All words you see ahead are those of the Diarists, with the exception of minor wording adjustments for clarity. I do edit for length, because often the Diarists have a lot to say. The Diaries are anonymous, and any fact that remains here is accurate: I have at times made details more vague, such as referring to a 'bakery owner' as a 'shop owner', simply omitting the names of identifying towns and establishments and, of course, changing all names.

You'll find that the Diaries are ordered, more or less, in the flow of relationships that adults experience. You will probably find yourself in most chapters of this book at some point in your life. Taken altogether, this book is a fluid portrait of people moving in and out of sexual and relationship ties over time – and a bit of a personal guidebook: it's fascinating to flip ahead and see what may be coming down the road for you or to read a Diarist similar to an ex and gain a new perspective.

The Diaries are not all flowers and daffodils. Some of these Diaries are lessons in *what not to do*, with Diarists making common blunders like never actually talking to their partners about their plans and needs. But overall, the Diaries are a joyous celebration of the diversity of sexuality and relationships. The happiest Diarists, without fail, enjoy the relationships that best fulfil their sexual and personal needs, often defying typical societal categories, and sometimes living quite stably in relationships far away from the dating-commitment-marriage-children-forever escalator that society ordains.

You are about to read the racy private lives of many people who may have made very different choices to your own. Every time you feel a wince, examine that feeling. You might find that you like the sting.

Arianne Cohen

EARLY IN THE RELATIONSHIP

1

IT'S SIMPLE:

I LIKE YOU, YOU LIKE ME.

the insecure cabaret dancer pussyfooting her way into a hot, healthy relationship

31, FEMALE, LONDON

THURSDAY

9:15 am: Awake, thinking about romantic chemistry. I trust my ex-boyfriend, and we still have a connection, but I don't have any depth of feeling for him, and I would still rather be in my loving relationship with my boyfriend of a few months. We both just left long-term relationships, mine of five years. I'm worried that this has made him wary of commitment (he was dumped); I'm also worried that I feel for him more deeply than he does for me.

5:35 pm: Spent the day shopping for costumes and make-up. Sounds glamorous, but it involved poking around in vintage shops looking for unflattering clothing like denim dungarees. Sometimes I wish the type of performance I do was sexier, but I know I'll never be the sort of person who can pull it off.

8:00 pm: Miss my boyfriend and would like to see him tonight. But I already emailed today and feel like I've reached my quota. He's had two discussions with me about needing space and wanting me not to contact him so much. I'd like to stress that I am not a constant contact sort of a person, never more than two to three emails or texts per day. But he doesn't want to feel he has to answer them. I know if he wants to contact me, he will. This only makes me realise that if he's not contacting me, he doesn't want to talk to me. This leaves me wondering why he doesn't want to talk to me, and why I feel that seeing each other once a week is not enough?

8:46 pm: It's quarter to nine and I'm wondering what my boyfriend is doing. I should be mixing music or emailing promoters, doing all the work I need to do, but right now I just wish he was here and fucking me.

9:32 pm: Feeling a little shamefaced. Got a text from my boyfriend asking to come over. Hormonal balance restored.

10:15 pm: I answered the door dressed as a boy, deep into rehearsal for a drag act. This was partly a test; if he freaked out then I'd have to seriously consider whether this was going to work. Fortunately, he's a performer too, and is as fine with boy-me as he is with girl-me.

10:32 pm: Became a girl again, and put on new lingerie. Definitely a win: lots of groping, breast squeezing and my favourite, nipple sucking. It's very flattering how sexy he finds my body, my breasts and arse in particular, and how vocal he is about it.

10:45 pm: We're talking about various options for tonight's pleasures. Him fucking me hard in the arse wins out. I love feeling his cock deep in my arse.

10:48 pm: He just said something interesting. We were talking about how we'd like to fuck, and he asked whether I prefer being on top with him in my arse, which we have tried in the past. I said I prefer on my front, and he asked whether that's because it's submissive. But in this case it's not. It's because I feel closer to him when his body is on top of me and encompassing mine more, and I feel a little exposed being on top, and more aware of my body, including the bad bits, which makes me far less likely to enjoy the sex and far less likely to come.

1:15 am: I gave him a blow job, then he lay me down on my front with my face pressed into the pillow and fucked me in the arse. I came quickly for me, after about ten minutes of intensive fucking, and my orgasm was amazing. I could feel him pulse inside me as I came, which made it even better.

1:20 am: Sleep. I'm finding him incredibly sexy tonight. I always do, but tonight he just seems more… powerful maybe? Masculine?

FRIDAY

10:00 am: Awake with just enough time to shower and get to a four-hour choreography session.

1:15 pm: Talking with a performer who is openly bisexual but married. Her sister has kids, and she envies her sister, but says that her sister has probably never experienced the kind of love she has. She says that I might meet the love of my life one day. I don't really believe in that. Unless that means I haven't met them yet? But how would I know? Instantaneously 'just knowing' that someone is the right person seems a bit implausible to me.

9:08 pm: Home to pack and go to boyfriend's. Damn, last night was good! We have such great, dirty, intense sex, the best I've ever had. I'm not sure whether it's because we're really suited to each other, or because I'm now in my early 30s and experienced enough to specify what I want. We do a lot of talking about what we want to do to each other before the fact.

9:38 pm: On my boyfriend's computer, noticing he has an email folder with his ex-girlfriend's name. (The page was open when I sat down!) Tempted to look? Of course! Going to? No way! Do I really want to know how amazing their sex life was/how beautiful he thought she was/how much he loved her? Nope. Especially as he's never texted or emailed anything remotely like that to me. And the vitriol he still expresses for her dumping him makes me think there are a lot of unresolved feelings there. I do live in a bit of fear that if she asked him back, he would.

10:54 pm: In bed at boyfriend's. He's playing computer games and I'm reading, which is perfectly fine with me. I'm seeing him for a second night in a row, which doesn't happen very often. Doubt we'll do anything sexual tonight as we're both tired, but cuddles will be wonderful.

SATURDAY

1:47 pm: Outside London for a show. Boyfriend has come with, which is nice as he hasn't ever seen me perform properly. He has his arm around me, and comments that I tuck under his arm (there's a seven-inch height difference), but that in fact he prefers to date women who are taller than him so they can put their arm around him. I am completely thrown, as there is nothing I can do about my height. Does this mean he'll eventually dump me when someone taller catches his eye? He says it 'doesn't mean he likes me any less.' This doesn't make me feel any better.

1:55 pm: I'm reminded of a night after a show he did a month back. He was chatting to a promoter's girlfriend who is this 6'3" gorgeous, intelligent and utterly lovely woman. I must have already known about his preference for tall women as I commented to another performer about it. I remember watching his face light up, and wondering if his face lights up like that when he talks to me? Crazy talk, I know, but it's small things like this that prey on my weird little mind.

1:59 pm: I'm always bemused when people talk about their 'types.' I only have two conditions: taller and older. The rest is negotiable. I'm worrying again that my boyfriend is with me only because he's flattered that I liked him so much, not because he actually fancied me.

10:05 pm: One act went well, one didn't, and I wanted to impress my boyfriend. Totally demoralising. He's a very honest person and he knows critique is helpful to me, so he told me what he thought. It will be useful when I get over feeling despondent.

1:07 am: Supporting another performer on the train home, assuaging her doubts. She's beautiful and incredibly talented and the bitchy part of me thinks she has no idea how good she has it. Why do I feel everything so hard?

3:00 am: Just home, so tired and worn out and despondent that I'm crying myself to sleep. Boyfriend does exactly what I need him to do, hold me and kiss my back and let me cry myself out. I can't articulate exactly what's wrong if I try, so it's the best thing to do.

SUNDAY

11:00 am: Still feeling despondent, but lots of chatting with boyfriend and some great sex has helped a lot. He's able to re-route my trains of thought.

11:15 am: Example: he was just playing with my large breasts. He loves feeling the weight of them and putting his face between them. I asked whether it was specifically my breasts he liked to do this to or he'd like to do it to any breasts in general. He stopped fondling and looked at me and told me he wasn't going to answer because he knew I was angling for the 'any breasts' answer, which would allow me to feel worse about myself. He was completely right. He saw straight through me and effectively snapped me out of myself. He is a treasure.

12:00 pm: More good sex, which involved him going down on me, me on him, him sliding four fingers into my pussy, lots of nipple sucking, me on top till he came, and him fucking me with a vibrator till I came. I love that we treat penetrative sex equally to all other sexual activities. We don't have just foreplay; everything is *play*.

6:12 pm: Didn't eat for 20 hours. Had something to eat and feel better but shattered. Happy I spent some time with boyfriend, who I probably won't see until next weekend. I'm worried that I'm leaning too much on my boyfriend at the moment. He says he understands, but previously he's said that he's not a bottomless pit of support and also (early on) that he liked the fact that I didn't need as much support as his previous girlfriends.

8:15 pm: The bed still smells of sex and him; this is very comforting. I am reminded of when my ex would come up and lie next to me and curl into me, just to be where I was for a while. There are days I'm certain he never loved me, because of how much he ignored me and was hurtful and verbally abusive, and because of how frightened I was of him toward the end when I moved out (it was only four months ago). And then I'll remember times like these and think maybe he did love me. I wonder if it was my fault for taking his love for granted?

8:23 pm: I hope my boyfriend and I can get to that same level intimacy. I'm getting better at being honest about how I feel (something I felt I couldn't do in my previous relationship for fear of the consequences), and he's getting better at explaining why he needs so much space.

11:00 pm: When I have a low self-image, I find I don't want to pleasure myself. Nor do I want my partner to do a selfless act (going down on me or finger-fucking me). When I'm feeling down about myself, I'll offer my breasts, my cunt and my mouth and any part of me he wants to use. It's more for the comfort of knowing I can please him, that I am useful and desirable in some way, even if I don't feel it about myself.

11:18 pm: No masturbating tonight I think, no matter how much Literotica.com I read. I enjoy reading erotic stories, although curiously, descriptions of overly 'hot' women will always put me off, because I can't relate.

12:08 am: Ended up doing so in desperation to try to get some sleep. It didn't work and it was quite depressing. At least one of my vibrators is reasonably quiet so it doesn't wake up the house. When I'm masturbating, I always imagine myself as thinner and prettier. I have a really deep-seated belief that I only deserve to orgasm when I reach a certain physical 'standard' (of my own devising). No idea where this came from, but it's hard to overcome.

MONDAY

9:51 am: Back at the boring day job, with all its lack of stimulus. Though I have got so randomly horny at work that I have to go to the bathroom and quickly bring myself to orgasm, there are no sexy thoughts today.

9:55 am: I think it would make a huge difference to my relationship if I was taller, as my boyfriend has mentioned he doesn't find short, plump girls attractive. Maybe if he didn't refer to the physical appearance of every girl we meet, I wouldn't be so paranoid about it. He's not sleazy. It's the level of honesty with which I'm having difficulties.

5:30 pm: Looking at a journal I kept with my former dom every time I disobeyed him. We met through work, and through a series of emails, established what we might be able to provide each other. We met up a few times. It was short and intense. The journal seemed important at the time. Now I realise how shallow it all was, how he just fulfilled a physical need that I thought was an emotional one: I thought that relinquishing to someone else's control was the only way I could gain any inner peace. It was an important lesson to learn, for me.

9:03 pm: Someone at Pilates told me that my life sounds so exciting compared to theirs. My life is full of clowns, strippers, jugglers and singers, and I'm so much happier for it. In my line of work, we sometimes take for granted the very fluid notion of sexuality. (I enjoy sex with women, but enjoy sex with men more.) Often we're okay about being in environments where various sexual practices are going on, without feeling uncomfortable about not getting involved. I know fetish models who aren't into BDSM, cross-dressers who are sexually straight, escape artists who aren't into bondage.

10:33 pm: A friend tweeted about a porn star she's currently obsessed with, and now I'm browsing online. I like porn. I first watched with a boyfriend when I was about 19. We fucked watching a hilarious Christmas-themed '80s vid with a dwarf actor called Short Studd. I find now that I watch most porn with the sound off, particularly European, as I can't stand how badly it's dubbed. I find a lot of porn definitely not to my taste, particularly those involving teenagers, but I have occasional fantasies about being a porn star.

TUESDAY

8:30 am: Conversation in the house today after one of my flatmates' boyfriends called her by a new name. My boyfriend calls me by a different form of my name, which I forget to respond to sometimes.

2:00 pm: Today is boringly standard. Meeting boss, more chat about my pending lay-off. Status on Kübler-Ross cycle: acceptance.

6:00 pm: I love my dance classes. Remembering a not-great ex who had a thing for dancers. One night he had a promotional pack of playing cards with pictures of dancers from the performing scene. He went through them going 'done her, dated her, snogged her, dated her'. *Why* did I date him?

6:02 pm: Oh yeah, I loved his house.

9:47 pm: Very tired after the dance class/run combo. I've run marathons in the past. In my line of work, thinner is definitely better. I defy any woman not to feel like a heffalump when surrounded on a weekly basis by the kind of women I am. They're so beautiful they take your breath away, and not in the slightly alien-catwalk-model way, but the kind of girl you see on the Tube and think, 'I wish I looked that way.'

11:41 pm: Although I miss my boyfriend a lot, not living together is a good thing for both of us as it gives us the time to concentrate on our passions. Work work work.

11:48 pm: I am way too tired for sex tonight. Although the thought of my boyfriend pinching my nipples is making me slightly horny. Not enough to masturbate.

12:06 am: Late-night text from my ex is knocking me. It isn't a booty call or anything sexual, just a friendly text to see how I am. I look him up on Twitter from time to time. At the end, dinners were quick and perfunctory, and he banned me from talking about the topics I love. (Yes, he actually asked me to stop talking about them, because he wasn't interested.) I stopped talking about myself at all. I hope my current relationship never gets like that. Yet despite everything I want him to be okay and happy. It's nice to know he cares.

WEDNESDAY

10:23 am: My ex sent another text last night that he misses me. I suspect he was drunk, and possibly just wants a girlfriend in general. I haven't loved him in a while, but I do still love him as a friend. He was a big part of my life for a long time.

10:28 am: I struggle to cope with how much space my boyfriend needs. I often think of him as several people, the worker (focused, doesn't like being bothered), the performer, the boyfriend and the solo person (the one I never get to see).

1:30 pm: Gah, bloody Facebook! Someone's tagged my boyfriend in photos with his ex. They're old, but I still felt my guts twist. When we started seeing each other he talked about her an awful lot and mentioned how stunning she is. Being pathetic, I looked up pictures of her on Facebook and admittedly couldn't actually see what he meant. In these photos she looks lovely. They look like they belong together in these photos. I wonder if he ever thinks we belong together. I haven't heard from him all day, and could use a hug.

1:44 pm: An email from the ex apologising for any hurt he's caused me. It does seem like he's worked through his anger at me leaving. I'm not sure what to write back. I'm not sure whether I should.

3:39 pm: Phone call from ex. It's nice to chat to him, catching up on what he's doing and what I'm doing. He says he's thought a lot about things over the past few weeks and wants to apologise. I didn't talk to him about my current boyfriend. I think he'd immediately be convinced that I left him for someone else.

3:50 pm: When he was talking to me he slipped and called me 'baby'. I thought, 'I'm someone else's baby now.' I hope that's true.

—⁓—

the madly-in-love 18-year-old hoping her relationship with an older bloke will survive uni

18, FEMALE, READING

WEDNESDAY

12:00 am: Woke up late today. Excited to go back to the place I first met my partner Jake. Should be fun. I am in a very happy, committed relationship with the loveliest man I have ever met. I know he is my forever; I just hope that I am his.

4:00 pm: Jake and I are at our first meeting place at an amusement park. It's where we had our first date eight months ago, but we met on a Facebook dating application before that, and spoke online for a month. I thought he didn't like me in person, so I went on a date with another guy, and there was no connection at all. I was being incredibly stupid letting Jake go. So we arranged a date and really clicked. Then he picked me up to go to his one evening, and then again the next, and following a little intimacy, we decided to be exclusive. I was so happy that I danced around on the phone to my best friend as soon as I got home!

4:15 pm: He brings up staying at his parents' holiday home. I take this as a rather large commitment, but perhaps this is normal for a long-term relationship. How would I know? I have no others to compare it to.

5:15 pm: Jake is talking about an ex. Once again I am green with jealousy. Will I ever get past my insecurities enough to know that he has everything he wants and more with me, and that no other woman will interest him more?

5:30 pm: Looking at myself in a bikini in a mirror. I can count nearly 100 imperfections. Jake can't find one.

7:00 pm: Dinner with Jake and my parents. I love that he fits in perfectly. It feels like he has always been here. He is going to university with me.

11:13 pm: In my room with Jake. He is playing Xbox. I keep thinking about my future with him, and although it seems bright, I find myself doubtful of whether he wants it as much as I do.

11:52 pm: He has just opened up to me about how much he is struggling. When he was younger, he had lots of friends, played football regularly for a good team, he was in a very successful band. But now at 23 he is doing a job he can't stand, and doesn't really have friends. At the moment I can't fix my own life, let alone his. If things keep going this way, I don't know if we will make it to university in September. Jake says I am the only thing keeping him smiling.

THURSDAY

11:40 am: Woke up late again. Missed morning class at college. Was having totally bizarre, hormone-driven dream about another woman. Although I know all women have them from time to time, I am completely freaked out and feel like a lunatic. There is no problem with my and Jake's sex life.

11:42 am: A big secret is that I used to be curious about bisexuality. It is something that both my parents and best friend are extremely disgusted by. So there was never anyone around that I felt I could tell. That is very much a thing of the past for me – a short, embarrassing chapter!

12:36 pm: Noticed that I have left a variety of things that I need for today at Jake's house. Ask him to bring them round. Realise that I always feel guilty when it comes to asking him for anything. Is that normal?

2:15 pm: Never do I feel less attractive than when I am in college. Saskia looks like a catwalk model, as usual. She's like me but with money and a nicer figure. We talk about my last relationship, with a melodramatic guy who dressed like a punk rocker and was clearly a little odd. It lasted a week and I dumped him for being too clingy. He tried to kill himself. Not good.

4:30 pm: In the park with best friend. She is a virgin and asks me some uncomfortable questions that proceed to make us laugh. I try to explain the complications of a relationship when sex becomes involved. Jake was my first sexual partner, and I am trying to adjust to a sex relationship. It still feels strange, and I am often uncomfortable with my figure around him. I started sleeping with him five months ago. We had been together two and a half months, sounds terrible to say in hindsight! But the timing seemed right and I was excited.

4:35 pm: I can't say there is anything sexual that I want to try. Everything is already very new and scary for me! I am happy with everything exactly the way it is. From what I hear from my girlfriends, I am very lucky to have a man who knows what he is doing. My parents allow him to stay over if we are going out clubbing, as it is about £15 cheaper to taxi back to mine than his, but he sleeps in the spare room. We always go to his house for anything physical, the only place we can really be alone.

6:00 pm: Home. Staying in my room as the idea of facing my parents over missing a class is daunting. I usually get along very well with my mum, but in the last few months, things have been starting to deteriorate.

9:45 pm: My 14-year-old brother is BLARING music from his room. He is treated brilliantly in comparison to me. Jake is furious as I fill him in on the latest inequality. He says he is struggling to not say anything as it is none of his business.

FRIDAY

2:30 pm: Spent most of my cashier shift daydreaming about going back to Turkey, this time with Jake. Very few fantasies of mine involve anything sexual, but rather moments of commitment and looking forward to spending the rest of my life with Jake.

4:00 pm: My daydream has shifted now, to a school reunion to show off the woman I have become since I was bullied and ignored at school. I would love to show them the person they missed out on.

6:30 pm: Parents come in to pick up a few last-minute purchases as the shop is literally closing. I am mortified! Pop off the till to ask them what they are thinking of for food. Dad says we are having 'chip shop chips'. I tell him for the thousandth time that I don't like them, and he proceeds to go ballistic.

7:00 pm: Text Louise to arrange to meet up on Tuesday to discuss important life updates – boys and gossip about the latest formed couples.

7:15 pm: In the car I find out that parents are not having chip shop chips, but in fact have bought themselves a microwavable Indian (quite the treat in our current hard-up financial times). It was simply me and my brother who were to have chips, and that was only because he wanted them. He is the favourite.

SATURDAY

10:29 am: Think happy thoughts about Jake. Every part of this relationship revolves around fun and seeing the other person smiling!

11:45 am: Mother and I walked to the local shopping centre with the dog to get some lunch – she even paid for mine and bought me a cake! We can get along so well sometimes. I think my mother is struggling to let go, and is not used to me being in a long-term, committed relationship. Jake and I can't do anything spontaneous or romantic, as we always have to run it past my parents first!

12:15 pm: At work and so far have spent all morning daydreaming about going back to Turkey with Jake and some uni friends, would be really brilliant! We have such similar personalities that I know we would enjoy it. Fingers crossed.

5:30 pm: Really pleased to see best friend. We now have a plan to get toned and fitter for my first and her second year of uni. I can't wait.

6:30 pm: Spoke to Mum about the possibility of going back to Turkey for a holiday in summer if our financial situation picks up.

She thinks it is a great idea for Jake to come along. He is ready, and so am I, but could it be a mistake?

6:40 pm: Hilarious image of Mum and Jake's awkwardness around each other in bathing suits. That moment is worth every risk.

SUNDAY

4:00 pm: *Very* glad to be leaving work. Had a new daydream for the second half of work. I was thinking I would love to do a school reunion when me and Jake are married, and preferably I am pregnant, so I can be like: 'HA! My life is amazing and none of you can do anything about it!' And I wanna be really pretty and stylish by then so I can laugh at their faces when they realise how stupid they were for ignoring me for five years – muahahah!

6:00 pm: Jake is coming over in a bit so I have been cleaning my room.

6:43 pm: Discussing rules and boundaries for uni again with Jake. We agreed that we won't see each other at all for the first two weeks as it is Freshers' and we need to be making friends. We should have separate friends so we can have time apart and keep our relationship as something separate from our uni lives, so that it is still something special. I'm keeping my fingers crossed that things will be fine. I know that I won't do anything to throw our relationship away, but what if he meets someone better?

10:01 pm: Going to bed, I am shattered. Jake has left me with a lot to think about and all I can picture is that if we break up at university, the pain of seeing him with another woman is going to kill me. Oh God, this has to work. I am still not 100 per cent in his feelings for me, despite constantly being told I am the one. How do you know?

MONDAY

8:30 am: Woke up feeling totally shattered. Managed to cycle the whole way to college and felt fantastic when I got here. Jake would have been proud, he cycles to work every day!

3:30 pm: Feel massively accomplished, cycled the whole way home and then two miles around town again. Started cleaning the house as a welcome treat for mother. Receive phone call from her giving me hell for sending a text to her instead of my gay friend. She delivers a lecture, then bans me from his flat and kills my mojo, therefore ruining my whole day. How does this woman have so much control on my life? Not. Happy.

5:00 pm: Best friend Aaliyah finally arrives. We again discuss the problems that me and Jake are having. He is currently working nights and I rarely get to see him for more than two hours before he has to go to work. He is depressed because all he does is work and sleep, but whenever I try to help him he makes excuses. He has to help himself a little, it is too much pressure for me to be the only thing in his life.

5:29 pm: Poor Aaliyah, being Muslim she is not allowed to date, but a half-Indian boy has been telling her he loves her for a long time, and she is not sure how she feels about it. Unfortunately he tends to be a bit of a 'player' and gets around a lot. He is also my ex from many years ago and I still hate him. Talking about him is always awkward.

10:00 pm: Well, this is my last entry. I am insecure about whether I will manage to keep Jake when we go to university together. I hope that Jake will allow me the opportunity to change and blossom into a more confident person.

—〜—

the sound engineer who can't think of anything besides his skinny-dipping, naked, vacationing girlfriend

31, MALE, BRIGHTON

THURSDAY

9:10 am: Just seen my girlfriend of three months off to Spain for the week. Tingling with longing, loneliness, anxiety, uncertainty.

9:51 am: Little bit calmer now. Cup of tea. Text her to apologise for being so intense; thus being more intense.

12:21 pm: Recording some lyrics. As much as I dread being without her, if I occupy myself, it's easier. I would write lyrics about her if it wasn't so close to the bone at the moment.

3:25 pm: Having a quick workout to shake the blues. Thinking about Essie constantly.

3:29 pm: I should mention I met Essie at my club job, and we've been seeing each other three months. Mustn't forget it's been a difficult couple of weeks. She had an abortion a week ago today – quite an early stage, so physically, at least, it wasn't bad for her. Neither of us had experienced that before. It brought us closer. I found it very sad and did weep on my own about the loss of a potential living soul. But ultimately I was quite glad of the opportunity to show her how supportive I can be. I started reading her *Northern Lights* by Philip Pullman. I'm a bloody nice guy, and attractive, and would be the perfect catch were it not for the crushing insecurity.

3:34 pm: Texted: *Hope you've landed safe and well.*

5:29 pm: Would absolutely love to get a reply but don't think I will, and wish I hadn't sent it. I don't think I've ever felt this much agony being in love with somebody.

5:30 pm: I'm sure I've said that before.

12:45 am: Spent the evening with my cousin Dev, and cycled six miles there and back. Not sure how many endorphins I need to balance out the anxieties. Missing her a lot.

FRIDAY

9:31 am: Woke up thinking how it sucks not waking up with Essie.

10:22 am: Alternating between playing with myself and determinedly racking my brain on what I need to do. Reach no concrete conclusions in 45 minutes. Need something to do in the daytime.

1:03 pm: I really wish I hadn't urged Essie to keep in touch. She was going to leave her phone at home, which shocked and panicked me. I also wish I hadn't cited that my urgency in this was from a bad experience with an ex, when she went away for two weeks and I only heard from her once.

1:05 pm: Off to work now. My ex is somebody who I'm not sure I'll ever quite feel finished with. Something went wrong with our sex life and it hurt me, I cheated on her, told her about it and we split up almost gradually over what felt to me like a year, and I do wonder how it may have changed if I hadn't cheated.

7:37 pm: I really hate my job – tonight is awful, soulless, abusive music at ear-damaging levels.

8:00 pm: Essie sent me a text saying that she was missing me and thinking about me lots. I want to cry. I don't know if she is protecting me or if she means it. Guess there's no need to torture myself – it's nice either way.

11:59 pm: Difficult shift tonight. An Eastern European girl called Sara is helping me. She is very quiet and smiley and made my missing Essie fade into the background. Though Jim, the giant bouncer, is getting on my nerves. It's because I've noticed him smiling at Essie. I can be so so so jealous.

SATURDAY

10:48 am: At least when I wake up thinking about cigarettes, I can hypothetically just go have one. I can't see her. Cigarettes and love: equally addictive.

10:50 am: Finding it very difficult to not feel inadequate or to compare myself to other men who appear to suit her better. Horrible habit.

10:55 am: It's also that she seems to be able to take it slower than I am able, which surely is an indication that she is not as taken with me as I am with her?

11:46 am: Just masturbated. Really good one. Fantasised about doing Essie outdoors, despite having Internet porn rolling in front of my eyes. I didn't find her that pretty when I met her. (I still don't, on a superficial level.) But her grace and demeanour and that calm, sexy voice are irresistible. I'm brainy, and I'm fairly sure I'd feel more secure in my relationship if I was more muscular.

1:50 pm: Dentist. Listening to the nurse and receptionist talk about how their boyfriends get jealous. Made me wonder if they're aware of beautiful souls like Essie.

8:04 pm: In work. Feeling sad. Need to get a different job. Essie pointed out to me that what I'm going to do for work doesn't have to be the same as what I enjoy doing. Sensible, that one.

11:00 pm: Just did a great blue-green lighting for a really sexy, voluptuous black girl dancer – amazing bum. Cabaret/burlesque. Good distraction.

2:00 am: Every time the floor manager looks my way, I try to catch her eye. Then I can't hold her eye because she's too gorgeous.

SUNDAY

11:23 am: Woke up feeling average, as often happens – neither excited, nor filled with dread. Think I need to become more interesting. A sure-fire way to do that is to become more interested in things.

12:00 pm: I've often suspected love and depression to be very similar. They're both overwhelming, debilitating and work in cycles. I truly feel that if you love something, you should be able to let it go, and

I'm wondering this morning if that is what I should do for Essie. She has a lot going on in her life.

1:13 pm: She took a bikini. Yeah. Not too thrilled by her parading her cute little body around. But it's just my imagination to be aware of. She told me she'd like to go skinny-dipping in summer, though, on the beach near where we live. Hope she means at night. I can't see me doing it.

5:19 pm: Watched the Grand National. Haven't thought a great deal about Essie, except for planning not to text her. Easier than I thought.

5:51 pm: Incredible how much music changes one's mood. In work, listening to lots of old school hip-hop. Brilliant. Perhaps I'm coming out of an Essie-obsessed daze.

10:09 pm: Text. She's been to a nudist beach where 'unfortunately' there weren't many nudists and she's burnt her bum. Not very happy about this. Best to not reply to that text.

10:18 pm: Oh come on. What the fuck does she expect me to say to that? If that is how she is, perhaps I'll soon find out that we're not right for each other. Perhaps she's drunk and not thinking. Fucking hate the idea of anybody else eyeing up her naked body. Well, I feel hurt.

MONDAY

11:32 am: Haven't replied to her text. Know I should text, 'Missing you, Sexy.' But need to consider how much the nudism bugs me first.

11:45 am: Nice phone call with Dev. One thing I've never told anyone is that my feelings for my cousin are very close to how being in love feels. I don't have any sexual desire for him, but I do love him so much that, in his company, I am rapt and in a bit of a daze. It doesn't make me feel tortured or gleeful. It just doesn't feel necessary to voice.

4:51 pm: Sent: *Missing you too, Sexy xx.* When she's back, I am going to ask her if she was nude on the beach. I don't think it's unreasonable to want her naked body to be for my eyes only. Is it?

6:49 pm: I'm reminded that we've only been together three months. Three days after our first date, we'd been having lots of sex, and then she cut me down and said she didn't want a relationship but she liked having sex with me and doing fun things. I was gutted. To tell the truth, our 'relationship' hasn't yet been qualified as anything beyond that.

7:02 pm: A few weeks ago she said to me that she was worried that I was getting ahead of her. (I was, and am.) And that she didn't want to be responsible for anybody else's feelings. I told her that I'm a big boy and I can handle my feelings. She liked that. I definitely think she's still a bit emotionally involved with her ex. I wonder if the nudist text was a test.

9:10 pm: Recorded some violin, ate dinner, watching a film now. I miss her. Just as I think that I'm happier on my own, I start missing her again. I truly hope she is re-thinking what I mean to her.

9:58 pm: I'd kill for a cigarette now. That nudist beach text.

11:17 pm: Sent a couple of explicit text messages just now to a girl I snogged once who's a complete tease. Just finished having a workout. Feel fairly rounded now.

11:19 pm: Texting has given me the means and temptation to be more lewd, suggestive and sleazy. I think it takes the sacredness and need for patience out of relationships. I've made a point of not adding my girlfriend on Facebook. I don't want to know what other blokes say to her or see the kind of photographs she posts or other people post of her.

TUESDAY

12:33 pm: With nothing to do in the morning, the late nights tend to creep up, even if since meeting Essie I have been a non-smoking, non-toking vegetarian (and, thus, full of life and spunk).

12:45 pm: Probably should text casual niceties, but they would feel like a lie. What I really want to communicate with her about is where I stand, and if she is as habitual a nudist as seems suggested.

2:01 pm: Text. This is a niggling detail but, particularly since she's been away, she never tends to ask me any questions in her messages. It does seem a bit like she's not interested or holding herself back from interest.

4:23 pm: Went to the park with a mate who's a mutual friend of ours. He's taller, fitter and more attractive than me. Fairly sure she has the hots for him and vice versa. How and why do we try to maintain relationships when there are so many obvious reasons not to?

5:43 pm: Just been chatting to an ex on Facebook. My heart skipped a beat when she suggested chatting on Skype. That relationship shaped up similarly to how my current one is. I was in awe of her figure, her composure, her vitality, her smile. I got so attached, and then in the end cheated because I felt so unloved. I won't ever cheat again. Cheating feels very exciting, and then absolutely terrible for years after.

7:12 pm: Texted: *I can't wait to kiss you.* But I can wait. Though I have this dull throb of longing for her, I feel a million times safer on my own. A lot less on edge.

11:59 pm: So she gets back early Thursday. I think I am looking forward to it. Been making music, not giving myself time to think.

WEDNESDAY

8:27 am: Want to masturbate, but am saving myself for her later. I want to pick her up and fuck her. I know I can just about do it. Not that she's heavy by any means. I did tell her a couple of weeks ago that I think women who are a bit overweight are sexier than those who are a bit underweight. First time I've seen her get pissed off.

8:34 am: I am battling various insecurities about the relationship, some of which spring from her being guarded and reluctant to tell me how she feels. I think I love her and I don't think she wants me to say it to her because I think she is still reeling a bit about her ex. Though this week has brought to light quite how fervent and irrational my jealousy can be, and how it springs from my oversensitivity.

12:03 pm: Work got cancelled. Sat on beach. Reckon my activities probably read like a guide to 'Why People Live in Brighton.'

12:20 pm: Talking to my mum. My mum is my first port of call for advice of any kind. I am trying to stop this being the case and at least create the illusion that I am more mature and less anxious (rubbish). Brought up Essie's naturist tendencies. Mum said she thinks my girlfriend's nudity is probably just an innocent expression of her freedom.

2:53 pm: So I'm now in my garden, essentially sunbathing but applying some intellectual gloss over my attempt to be sexier for Essie in the form of reading a science book.

7:53 pm: Really, really want to masturbate but am resisting. I've got to shrug off the nudity thing and just be nice tonight. To be loved you have to be lovable.

—*w*—

the counsellor in a week-long gay relationship, wondering whether to ditch his cybersex buddies

41, MALE, MANCHESTER

WEDNESDAY

10:47 am: Text from my new boyfriend Luke, saying that he can't stay over tomorrow after all. What a surprise. I shouldn't be this cynical, since we officially got together last week. We've known each other for seven years, and have had the odd fling, but we've never got into a relationship. He's keeping me at arm's length.

4:00 pm: My job requires me to spend the middle of the week a couple of hours away. I stay over some nights, which is a bit of a bind, but not really an issue for hook-ups, as there is always Grindr (gay hook-up networking, surely one of the most revolutionary apps in the App Store). Going home tonight, though.

8:27 pm: Back. My usual online contacts are tapping me up for a cyber-wank on-cam. I'm a very attractive gay man: lean and toned, and look like I'm in my late 20s. By all accounts, I am pretty good in bed. But frankly, I am too tired for cybersex tonight.

8:28 pm: Though there is this really fit Newcastle lad, 19 and very keen.

9:15 pm: Taking stock of my sex life. In the last two weeks I have slept with: a very sexy 32-year-old; a really beautiful ex, 24, who has HIV (we are amazing in bed together; he's a friend with favours);

Harry, a particularly horny 17-year-old who I have been tracking on Fitlads.net for the last year, where he's masquerading as an 18-year-old; and Luke, though we haven't actually had sex yet (he says I'm too big for him – I am only eight inches, for God's sake!).

9:20 pm: Truth be told, Harry was the best of the lot (amazing body, amazing blow job, loved being rimmed and, after initial misgivings about how big I was, absolutely loved being fucked). When I was 18, my first gay experience was with a 40-plus man.

9:22 pm: Phew. It makes me think. Who's in charge here, me or my cock?

12:00 am: Going through my porn collection. I belong to a porn club, where a guy records it and I get new batches in.

3:15 am: Well, I'm up wanking to what's left of my porn collection. Why? Mainly because most of it was shit, not much took my fancy, and I just trawled through what was left, and by the time I was in a position to orgasm it was like past 3am.

THURSDAY

8:24 am: First thought when I woke up this morning: Text Birger and Harry, as they are both wanting a threesome with me tomorrow. Sigh. I met Birger on Fitlads. We have been fucking for a year or so now. He's very beautiful, could be in better shape, massive cock, though. Hmmmm.

8:27 am: I should say that I am not usually happy when people describe me only in terms of my cock.

3:25 pm: One half of the threesome is in place. Birger.

6:17 pm: Harry hasn't texted back. Will I go through with it? Would it be fair to Luke? That's the question.

8:00 pm: Getting ready for Luke coming over. I'm going through that relationship period when you're not sure if the relationship is going to happen. Feeling ambivalent, mainly because I am just not sure how into me the object of my attention is. I have been chasing him for like eight years now (his excuse always was, 'I don't want to hurt you – I'm crap at relationships,') and I finally persuaded him last week to say yes.

9:16 pm: Threesome is on. Harry has responded positively. And my fella is here. Mmmmmm.

12:15 am: Really lovely night with Luke. He was generally touchy-feely, and said all the right things, like, 'I'm not going anywhere.' Nice.

FRIDAY

7:38 am: Luke is so sexy with his smooth skin and ample cock. Except no sex this morning: he's in too much of a rush to get himself sorted for work. Grrr. That, in turn, means the threesome tonight is on. Just this time. I'll justify my dalliance by the fact it's on the cusp of our getting together and had kinda been organised.

8:57 am: The threesome is off. At my behest. To be honest, I think Luke has done enough to convince me that he is serious – even if he *did* dash to the loo as I was sucking him off this morning. A threesome just wouldn't feel right. So I texted Harry and Birger. My conscience is clear for the mo.

3:00 pm: I feel a little frustrated that Luke didn't see me right, sexually, this morning.

9:55 pm: Taking stock of my relationship life. There's a certain type of person I have a tendency to go for who sets off insecurity in me. A sustained bout of therapy seven years ago taught me that. The trick is to not go for that type of person again. I don't *think* Luke's that type. I need a soulmate and companion. Not a mental health problem.

2:19 am: Well, I am about to go to bed – haven't even had a wank today, and I am not horny in the slightest right now either. Even if one of my cybersex buddies showed up on MSN right now, I'm not sure whether I would be up for a wank. Strange for me. I have a massively high sex drive that keeps me going back.

SATURDAY

10:53 am: Packing for holiday, a week in Eastern Europe, woohoo. My ex will be there, Goran, the love of my life, and some friends.

11:15 am: Am still angling for a nice wank before I go, but my libido is firmly AWOL right now. I'm not sure why. Possibly Luke has got to me?

11:45 am: Sent Luke a sexy text last night. He ignored it. Maybe I feel a bit rejected. He does this every time I send one.

2:39 pm: Email from Goran about travel details. We still feel a lot for each other. He's a stunningly beautiful guy who nurtured and loved me from the moment we met. We spent five years together, but the fact is, you have to play the hand you're dealt, and everything was perfect, except the sex. I loved him so much, made it work, with an open relationship and Viagra whenever I was with him. We almost got married, and finally split up to my eternal regret eight months ago. I miss him terribly. Though it was the right decision. Sometimes you click sexually, and sometimes you don't, and that was the long and short of it. I will love him forever.

2:41 pm: Relationships all have their shelf life, and you enjoy them while they last. Life-long relationships are the exception.

3:00 pm: Boyfriend has been in touch: he was at a funeral, and is not feeling too good. Will miss him while I travel, and will certainly miss his beautiful body and cock, mmmmm.

3:57 pm: Spoke to Luke, and he was cool. I am beginning to realise that his relaxed attitude is just that – a relaxed attitude. It doesn't mean that he isn't serious about us. There comes a point where you realise that the relationship is serious enough to head down that monogamy path.

4:11 pm: All packed and ready to go, less that wank I promised myself.

5:15 pm: You know how there is good sex and bad sex? Well there is also good wanking and bad wanking. The last hour was an example of the latter: trawling around on Gaydar chat for someone to cam with, settling for someone I didn't particularly fancy. You see the person on camera and you wank, and it's shit. Oh well, at least that's done and won't be on my mind. Not sure of the holiday opportunities for wanking or sex.

12:36 am: Sent Luke a text outlining how I feel about him. It said: 'I feel a lot for you. I have no idea what you're feeling.' No reply as usual. He really is crap at responding. And he doesn't text at all unless I do. I don't know how to play this really. I'll work something out.

1:14 am: Holiday tomorrow. Maybe I can put all the fretting about this new relationship behind me… maybe.

SUNDAY

6:28 am: Holiday today, smiling all over. No text back from Luke, which bothers me. His propensity to just ignore my messages has me wondering all sorts: does he still like me? Does he care? Is he about to dump me? Etc. All the usual teenage stuff. Gonna put it out of my mind.

1:08 pm: At the airport, reliving how I met Luke. He was very young (just 18, eight years ago) but very emotionally bright and very taken with me. We had a passionate kiss in the front of my car and a grope (that's when I first felt that perfect cock that, so many years later, makes me go weak at the knees). But somehow it never happened, much as I tried. He evaded and evaded me and then denied me and then moved abroad.

1:16 pm: On my flight, and feel slightly sad because, as happened last weekend, I haven't heard a peep from Luke. Well, not since we spoke yesterday morning anyway. It's like he disappears into a communication black hole on the weekends. I wonder, is this something we need to talk about?

4:15 pm: Spent the flight thinking about how Luke promised me the sex of my life when we finally get round to it. Turns out he's more top than bottom these days, which I am too, but am willing to compromise in his case and go fifty-fifty. I need some action.

9:05 pm: Finally got hold of Luke. My iPhone has gone tits up, not receiving any texts. Luckily this hotel has Wi-Fi chat. Luke said that he finds it hard to open up until he's comfortable. Well, that explains a lot and really helps me. So the compromise is: he tries to tell me more to help me, and I try to calm down. The whole gay relationship thing: sorted!

12:05 am: Back from chatting with a really sexy, very intelligent, gorgeous guy who I was flirting with at a stag do a couple of weeks ago. I've known him for years, but he had a long-term boyfriend. Our drunken chat had me flirting outrageously, and he seemed receptive to the idea, so I suggested a foursome with him, his boyfriend and Goran, who's arriving here very late tomorrow.

12:15 am: I just told him, 'Fuck it, why don't you and I just get it on?' His response: 'I would, but I'm not sure how I'd explain it to my fella!' Not exactly a ringing rebuff. Though it makes me think: am I in charge, or are my urges?

MONDAY

9:00 am: First day of holiday, thinking how lucky I am to even be here. Here meaning both 'on holiday' and 'alive.' My ex almost gave me HIV. When we first got together, we got tested and then had sex unprotected. We stopped going out, and this one time we ended up shagging. He got the positive result some weeks later. I went for three months waiting for my results.

12:48 pm: Sweet text from Callum. He was the love of my life for a while. I met him when he danced over, one loved-up night at a club. It was a love-at-first-sight thing. He had a lovely lithe body and perfect cock and was just really *willing*, as you would expect from a horny 19-year-old. We were on-and-off for seven months, and my heart was properly broken for the first time, precipitating an emotional breakdown on my part. We have remained close, though, and had many dalliances. I have to say, our friendship has only really taken off since we both stopped the whole sexual contact thing.

2:31 pm: Ha ha ha, most amusing. My mate Rob was just taking me through the latest iPhone gay social-networking apps. Seems there's a whole world out there that I still need to hook into. He and his civil partner have a colourful sex life (threesomes, saunas, the like). I am jealous – they have the security of their emotional attachment, and they've allied all the perks of playing the field: wow! I want some of that.

2:36 pm: Thank God for technology. In my 20s, I mainly used a gay phone line to get off.

3:38 pm: In my hotel room, trawling online. I have profiles at Gaydar, Fitlads. I will only shut them down when I am sure things are solid with Luke. Hedging maybe? Damn right!

10:15 pm: Out on the town. Luke messaged me and was so caring and attentive. He even said at the end, *It's my job to make you happy because I'm ur fella.* Which is such a sweet thing to say. So the whole thing is looking more and more promising. Things he is saying give me warm feelings inside.

12:30 am: Got back from town in the early hours to find messages from this guy here on Grindr, which amused me. Not sure how I feel about going to see him while my ex is arriving here tomorrow.

12:40 am: I miss Luke.

2

TOGETHER. FOREVER?

the construction guy with a penchant for hookers, and a girlfriend none the wiser

39, MALE, HERTFORDSHIRE

WEDNESDAY

5:50 am: As usual, I woke up with a tent in the duvet. A bit sleepy-eyed, but horny all the same. My partner of two years is dead to the world. I could run the bed through a car wash and she would keep sleeping.

5:55 am: Up and into the shower. I catch a glimpse of myself and think, 'Not bad.' In hindsight, my big ears have been a godsend, really. For all the trouble I have had with women – and there has been quite a lot – had I been a Brad Pitt, there would have been even more problems.

6:33 am: Train journey. It's the same four people in the carriage every day. The other three have been zombiefied, and I have given up saying hello. Funny, I am confident in work, but I fear rejection when it comes to the ladies. I have real trouble telling them I fancy them. Eye contact is a no-no unless I have them at home, or have seen them no end of times. For example, the lovely lady at the supermarket. I can flirt with her all day because she has no choice but to engage, and I am positive she looks forward to our exchanges.

7:28 am: As most mornings, a little bit of banter with the boys. Amazingly, everyone outside of me thinks I am happy-go-lucky.

And you know? I suppose on the outside I would think that of myself too.

8:48 am: Just saw one of the girls on site, the Hot One. She is sooooo hot I go weak at the knees when I see her. An explosion of fireworks goes off in my tummy, mind and loins all at once.

1:35 pm: Work, work, work. I sent a little romantic gesture to my partner today – some chocolates and some new sexy underwear – and even though it was sweet, it will result in nothing. I don't know how much longer I can take the constant rejection. Who knows when my monogamy belt will break? I wanted to remain faithful but feel I won't be able to.

4:31 pm: What an afternoon: a young lad rushed off to hospital. An accident kinda wakes you up a bit. You ask yourself, why am I moaning about me? Though I am sure tomorrow I will be back to asking why I'm not getting sex and attention.

8:00 pm: Getting a drink with the girlfriend on the way home. We bumped into an ex of hers and the flirting started. Ummmmmmmm. Now how come I don't get that flirting any more? For fuck's sake, it has only been two years. I thought we're in the honeymoon period, but that must only be me.

9:30 pm: As the alcohol flows, my sense of rejection and hump are dying down. Am I just getting used to this, or is this the way it goes? Would I be better off on my own? I'm frustrated, but good at hiding it.

10:30 pm: Not an unpleasant night, but find my eyes wandering behind her back to all the women in the bar, wondering, 'What if?'

11:45 pm: Just got in. All I want to do is shower and sleep. My partner wants to drink and chat.

11:50 pm: It really is all about her. I have become weak in this relationship and am feeling like I am worthless. I have convinced myself no more naughty breaks in London or romantic breaks in the Cotswolds until I have tackled this. All don't woo the woman any more.

THURSDAY

8:34 am: At work again and looking forward to seeing the Hot One. I get to have her on my rounds today. Harmless but meaningful for me. She enjoys the attention, but is clearly not interested in me, but I do like to make her blush.

10:31 am: About to spend an hour with the Hot One. Ate breakfast. Butterflies on a full stomach – not a good call. Crush is definitely the best way to describe my feeling towards her.

11:00 am: Just seen the Hot One. Time for me to pop off and have some Man Time thinking about her again. Damn she makes me horny. I only have to see her from one side of the room, and instant erection. And this time it's one of those that just won't go away so I will have to deal with the bugger instead.

11:22 am: Back. I fantasise about the Hot One a bit, but not as intensely as an encounter the other week: this woman will be in my heart for the rest of my life. Shame she lives thousands of miles away and I will never see her again.

12:40 pm: The Hot One came over and my heart skipped. Oh my god, she has no idea how I much I like her. She suggested I join the gang for a drink tonight and, well, how could I refuse? If only she could tell that I like her and be responsive too.

1:26 pm: We had a giggle on our rounds, but I have to stop and just ignore the Hot One from now on. She is in no way interested. Get a grip, man.

1:42 pm: Feeling horny as hell, and a girl at work caught me looking down her top today. She's now wearing a scarf.

2:52 pm: Made a boo boo this morning my taking the car, and now have to forgo the night out as the girlfriend is complaining. Depressing thing is, she will be asleep by 9 pm. I will be sat in front of shitty TV until silly o'clock eating away at myself. I wouldn't be so frustrated if she was a little more lively and, well, sexy-acting too. She is not extremely good-looking (I tend to settle for average-looking women, and fear the good-looking ones), but she oozes sexiness and is just lovely.

4:15 pm: Work work. I am a dirty little devil at work. I would say that 90 per cent of the numerous women that I've dated, slept with or had one night/day stands with have been at work. In offices, in houses, in hospital, in all sorts of environments. I have been somewhat a tart all my life. If I had of been better looking, I would of been unstoppable.

4:37 pm: I have always wanted to sleep with a lady boy. I am totally heterosexual but I find it incredibly erotic: a chick with a dick. I wouldn't marry one, but I would sleep with one, and would probably let one fuck me too, as I like my butt being played with – not something I've found most women like to do. In fact, I am at my desk at work getting the hardest boner as I write this, and have just seen The Hot One at the same time. Tis a good feeling.

5:45 pm: Got in from work, knowing well, by the exchange of emails, that sex is yet again not going to happen. So I have a choice: nip out to the supermarket via the whorehouse, or go online and do some masturbation. I reckon I can't afford a prostitute today, so online it is. Funny because when I am masturbating, I am obviously in the zone and it's all good, but after, I feel like, 'Was it worth it?' And then I'm annoyed that I have to wank so much and don't get any physical attention. I can't begin to tell you how much I would love the feel of a mouth around my cock right now.

5:48 pm: I could go to the whorehouse and get one, but it's more than that: it's feeling like the person doing it *wants* to.

8:00 pm: Just got to a mate's house for drinks, drugs, loud music, backgammon and Scrabble. A weird combination, but we get to chat rubbish and then are numb to it the next day. My girlfriend is out too. If it were Friday, I would be out much later and have the urge to call in a couple of hookers. But I'm meeting my girlfriend on the way home.

10:30 pm: Met my girlfriend out, and we're now on the train. My girlfriend hasn't had as much to drink as I thought she would of, and is touchy-feely. A nice change, to be honest.

11:15 pm: We just showered, and I thought, 'Whoop whoop, we might get it on tonight!' So I started to caress her, and in seconds she was, 'No no, I'm tired.' Of course my heart dropped and I got annoyed.

11:18 pm: Times like this, I wonder how the woman can love me, and yet not lust after me at all? It don't matter how much she says, 'It's not you.' I *must* be part of it. If I was still *the one*, she'd feel it from time to time. I mean, if she went on all fours and just ooh-ed and aah-ed a bit, it might feel like she wanted me for once.

11:35 pm: Downstairs, logged into PornHub.com. This is my way of trying to steer away from going out tomorrow night and either booking a hooker or pulling some girl into a hotel. I, like any man, like the odd off-the-cuff thing in real life. You know: anal, squirting, roleplay. But due to the lack of enthusiasm I normally encounter, it usually ends in a porn substitute.

12:15 am: Had two or three wanks. What I really crave is just someone who wants to come on to me and give me a blow job from start to finish. It's amazing how something so simple can make a man feel entirely wanted and gratified. Not all the time, but I haven't had this for years.

12:25 am: The irony is that when I do pay for a hooker (at least three times a week nowadays, though some weeks I do without) that is all I want, but I can't ask for it because it defeats the reason for getting a hooker. A transaction is not the same as having someone wanting to please you. Going to sleep on the sofa.

FRIDAY

5:50 am: Awoke on the sofa, another wank.

7:37 am: As I head to 40, I should really take a step back and worry about me for a change. Do the things I have put off for years. I would like to explore several things I have not. I find the fact that women can squirt amazing, and would love to see, taste and enjoy the experience. But 'Hi, my name is _____. Do you squirt?' doesn't really work. I have dabbled in anal sex and enjoy it but, without sounding arrogant or anything, I have a larger and thicker-than-normal cock, and every girl that has said that anal is okay has done it once or twice, and then shied away.

12:00 pm: Thinking about last Friday. I had popped a pill, had a few lines and was on a nice lush high, laughing, taking the mickey out of the group, a really nice vibe. From the corner of my eye was this American girl. She was soooo stunning that I first I could not engage in conversation. Then her other group disappeared, and she asked if she could join us.

12:05 pm: Now, she was 23 – half me – a subconscious barrier to deter me from coming on to her. Off we all went clubbing. As soon as the first song came on, she shook what her mama gave her. The two of us were grinding and dancing. Now, I do this with a lot of girly friends, because I am one of the few men they will let it all go with on the dance floor. I didn't see our connection. More smoking, chatting, a few more lines, another couple of clubs, then back to my mate's place. She was wearing my coat and holding my hand. We sat together, she was cold and snuggled against me. Still I didn't realise. I have so many female friends young and old, and it's not abnormal for me to be close to a girl platonically. Around 5 am, she mentioned twice that she should leave. I hailed her a cab and put her in. The cab drove 10 feet and stopped, she jumped out, ran back and kissed me with the power of one million kisses. She then kissed my nose and ran back into the cab and was gone forever. I have never felt so alive, ever.

12:15 pm: Sitting at my desk, kicking myself for not seeing the signs earlier. But I'm grateful it was as special for her as me.

8:00 pm: Out with some of the crew to a local pub. The Hot One is here. Last time we went out, she told me about a drunken session where she kissed one of the other people at work. It was a secret, but the guy did generously tell me about it. I was gutted. Now she's telling me about it too, and I'm trying not to react. She says, 'If you had been there, it would've most likely been you.'

11:12 pm: Making sure The Hot One is home safe, and she invited us into her place. I had a brief look: Very homely, very clean, and I had to get out of there as my imagination was running a marathon.

11:40 pm: Home. The girlfriend has a raging hump. At the beginning it was like a firework display – inside, outside, upside down. She's a really nice girl, and I've had more fun socially in the last two years than in the previous dozen with my ex, because my new girl lets me spread my wings. She makes me happy socially, but sexually it's like being with an old sack of spuds.

11:55 pm: In the back room again, and my thoughts are totally on The Hot One, incorporating all the new things I heard and seen. Me and The Hot One will have some special time.

12:33 am: More porn, more masturbation, almost in spite this time, and off for a joint. If only I had a few quid behind me to go off like a younger man, let my beard grow and fish off the back of a boat, drinking rum and having fun with native girls, and just saying, 'Conformity and work? Fuck ya.'

SATURDAY

5:15 am: More special time with The Hot One in the spare room.

6:15 am: Hung-over, so two pints of pomegranate juice.

11:52 am: Today we have people coming for dinner for 21 different tapas dishes, so it's off to the supermarket. There is still an air of 'you twat' coming from the girlfriend and I don't know why.

4:00 pm: Still feeling fuzzy-headed. Hair of the dog. But cooking and prepping, music, ass shaking. In my element.

7:00 pm: Dinner guests here, I've drunk a couple of jägerbombs. Wine is starting to flow, the new guy is really nice.

8:30 pm: My girlfriend is not a very good drunk. I find her constant repetition, loudness and lack of breaks annoying. In fact, I more than dislike it.

9:45 pm: She just brought up my lateness and why she's pissed at me. Her example: Last week she was horny and decided she would make an effort for me when I came home, and dressed in some uniform of sorts. Now, this was after *soooooo* long of her not coming on to me. Now, I am no mind reader, and if with current technology, she had suggested that I leave and come home now, I would've. But because I came home a tad later than planned, she got the hump.

9:48 pm: It's been a mostly shag-free year, so how the hell am I supposed to know?

1:00 am: After they all left, another barney, mostly due to too much booze. Another night in the other room. I see a pattern now. I really think it's time I lived alone.

SUNDAY

6:00 am: Hang over for the other half. I'm downstairs and starting the deep clean. Never thought I would see the day, but now have started to enjoy cleaning. Music on, sun shining, ass shaking – I am becoming a domestic god.

9:34 am: The other half got up and starting criticising the washing. I said, 'You know what, pisshead? Fuck you.'

11:34 am: Not proud of this. I normally respond in a more productive and less aggressive manner. The rest of the morning spent sharing sarcastic comments.

1:15 pm: Out for a drive, enjoying the sunshine and music in the car.

3:48 pm: On the drive back swung into a massage parlour and had the most lovely Thai girl walk over my back and suck and fuck me like it was going out of fashion. Then she washed me, dressed me up again and kissed me on my merry way.

3:50 pm: Do I feel guilty for this? Hell no. I have actively used escorts and whores when the mood takes me since I was a teenager, mostly when I am drink-and-drugged up.

7:30 pm: Just finished dinner, and have been accused of being half-hearted with the housework. For fuck's sake, I wash the clothes, the pots, the pans. I vacuum, polish, mop and clean, I do the DIY. Far more than her. I have become a slave.

8:32 pm: You know, I have clocked up a good understanding of women. I have had hundreds of one-night stands and short affairs. Once I cross the threshold and have been welcomed in, I feel at home and don't even realise I'm flirting. This is when I shine and things go well all the way. I now see that I'm a kind, generous, loving, kinky, sexy, horny man with a heart of gold. I know my personality is my gift, and that I can fit in any environment with any class of people. But what I didn't realise is that I'm a pushover and weak. I worry about other people's feelings before mine, and then whinge to myself when none of my needs are met.

11:00 pm: Spent the rest of the night on my PC watching films like *Last Boy Scout, Armageddon, I, Robot, Avatar*, and playing Xbox while the Grumpy One watched chick flicks and soaps all night. Doesn't really bother me, as we have an immense clash of box viewing.

11:05 pm: More and more I realise that I'm living with my best mate/mum. I will miss this diary, as I have found it very therapeutic.

—w—

the drama queen over-analysing and melodramatising her relationship to death

27, FEMALE, MANCHESTER

TUESDAY

6:30 am: Sam's alarm going off, still set from last week. Of course he slept through it.

8:10 am: Sam left. Now I lay here thinking, should I just confess to him that I feel sad we're not spending our Easter weekend together as planned, or leave it? Now he's going to visit his family for two days, smack bang in the middle, and I have to wait around hoping he'll spare me some time.

8:12 am: I ring him; he's driving.

8:30 am: By the time he calls back I chicken out. Why ruin his day?

1:52 pm: Just been on the phone to Sam. We met in the US when we were travellers, when he followed me across the country hoping to sweep me off my feet. And so he did. Now six months in I find issues arising daily. He has been supporting the two of us while I've been looking for a job, so I feel guilty. (My new job starts in two weeks.) Plus Sam was diagnosed with a neurological illness three years ago. He feels every moment is precious. And cuddling and staying in is not enough for him. Planning holidays must feel like the silliest idea.

1:54 pm: I'm sat here thinking about the future with a knot in my stomach. It's either going to be amazing or we're both going to be miserable. Which will it be?

4:00 pm: Excited about date night, something I thought we should try after I realised that work, gym, football and cricket all took time out of our (well, his) schedule. Showered, shaved my legs, smothered myself in body butter. Date night ends in date sex, right?

4:10 pm: Our sex life is always up and down in terms of quantity. He has a sex drive; I just think he doesn't want to have sex with me at times. It's led me to feel insecure about myself, my body, and caused me to have serious self-esteem issues.

6:20 pm: He just came home. I was surprised, as he always goes to the gym. I think my saying, 'What are you doing here?' wasn't quite the reaction he was looking for! Downhill from there. He was instantly in a bad mood, quiet.

6:45 pm: Just found myself lying on the bed with him, and he confessed that the last four days have been miserable for him because all he can think about is that when we met and were just friends, he heard me having sex with a guy we were staying with. That was six months ago, yet it doesn't make a difference. He still punishes me for it. I think he always will. I am keeping my cool and carrying on getting ready.

7:00 pm: We made it to the front door, and then he chose to walk straight up the stairs to the bathroom. I went back to the bedroom, and the argument got out of control. Well, I talked and he stayed quiet. I decided to pack my things and go back to to my parents' house.

8:25 pm: He watched me pack, call a taxi and walk out in the rain. I am smoking. I'd stopped smoking when I got together with Sam; he hated the smell. But I feel numb. Is he going to just let me walk out? We've had arguments before and I've packed, but I never actually wait. I am stood here waiting for a taxi!

8:30 pm: Sam just came outside and stared at me. I hate the fact that he just stands there and doesn't fight for us. Why am I the only one so passionate about what we have? I told him to stop standing there staring, so he got in his car and left. And I'm in my taxi to the train station.

8:40 pm: I was half expecting him to be here, waiting to stop me, but he isn't. He sent a text, though, saying that the reason he has a go at me sometimes is because he wants me to be the person that I was when he met me, full of energy and life. Not the slob that sits at home and does nothing.

8:48 pm: I rang him. He was very quiet, so I asked him why he hadn't asked me to stay. He said he wanted me to stay and had said it every other time.

9:30 pm: Sam met me at the train station, with tulips. He thinks they're my favourite flower. I don't know why; they're not. I don't have the heart to tell him that, though.

10:02 pm: We talked in the car. Well, again, I talked and he said very little. I was angry. If I was such a slob and so unmotivated, how had I found an amazing job? How is it that our place – sorry, *his* place – is always clean with fresh bed sheets every week? How is it that his lunch is made for him, and dinner on the table?

10:15 pm: The outcome: he decided he would change his approach. How? I don't know.

11:00 pm: We end up sitting in bed, eating and watching Japanese anime. I realise we're not having date sex. He's hugging me and has a boner, but it's not going to happen. I stopped getting excited every time he got an erection a long time ago. What's the point if he probably just thinks about me with other guys when we're having sex?

WEDNESDAY

8:07 am: Sam has just left for work. This morning was normal. He'd said to me last night that he doesn't want me to get up and make him breakfast. But this morning I did, otherwise he wouldn't have time to eat anything.

8:58 am: Just texted Sam and asked him why he didn't try making a move on me last night. Is it because he doesn't fancy me anymore?

9:08 am: Ten minutes, and he still hasn't replied. Maybe he'll just ignore that too.

9:01 am: He's emailed me a poem:

> *I want it so badly I need it even more*
> *Without it very sadly*
> *The future a mighty bore*
>
> *I have dreamt of it so long*
> *I have felt it in my grasp*
> *The feeling so strong*
> *To let out a quick gasp*

I will never give up I will cherish forever
The love of my life
Which nobody can sever xx

9:05 am: That's the poem Sam just emailed me. I'm liking the use of initiative but I still want to know what it is that stops him from being physical with me. I've never had this problem before. My ex and I used to have a 'shag night' at least once a week. Hours and hours of lovemaking. This isn't right. When I'm middle-aged, have kids and don't have time, then fine.

3:04 pm: Just had a bit of an argument with Sam. He's constantly on all his friend's Facebook pages, leaving them messages. I can't remember the last time he's written on my wall. Drives me crazy. But not just that, he'd had a picture of the two of us as his profile picture and today he changed it to a goofy picture of himself. That kinda threw me over the edge.

10:53 pm: Dinner with my friend. I'm wondering why I'm even in a relationship.

11:40 pm: In the spare room upstairs. I was lying in our bed with so many questions going through my mind about this whole relationship and just crying. Sam didn't understand what was going on and the poor guy just got abuse hurled at him from me. I grabbed a pillow and went to the spare room.

12:38 am: Still in the spare room. He came upstairs to bring me back down. But we carried on fighting and I ended up coming back up. He got really angry and called me a drama queen, and said if I go, he won't ask me to come back, and that his illness makes him tired. Guilt treatment.

THURSDAY

7:15 am: Crept back into bed with him at 6:30 and hugged him. He ignored me, and just got up like normal.

8:15 am: We didn't talk until he came downstairs, when I asked why he had said his illness was affecting him. And why should I not be kept in the loop? I'd be the one who'd have to look out for him if he got bad. He said that if he went past some stranger on the street who was crying, he'd feel more for them. My tears don't mean anything because I cry all the time. Why doesn't he realise that it's because he *makes* me cry? He asked me if I would be here when he got back. I didn't know what to say.

8:17 am: I ask if he's going to kiss me goodbye like he always does. He says he doesn't want to. Peck on cheek. He left.

8:18 am: I grab a towel (I'm not dressed) and run to the door, but he's gone. Call him three times, and when he answers, ask why he didn't want to kiss me. He replies that he doesn't want to kiss someone who was about to leave him.

8:50 am: Sam just called from work. He says two things: Firstly, it's not a bad thing that he always pushes me to go to the gym. (I've gained 14 pounds in the last six months.) And secondly, he will be going away for the weekend in a couple of weeks to Portsmouth to visit his friends. One of them is an ex-girlfriend. Great! How do I feel right now? Numb. Because I'm about to ruin something that could have been great.

12:53 pm: Just awoke again. Sam's not answering my calls.

2:06 pm: Spoke to Sam very briefly; he says he's been busy at work. Everything is weird; I don't know why I'm still here. But this whole thing is my fault; I started it. Sam thinks that one day we'll magically be okay. He doesn't realise that we have issues to work through, and if we don't we might as well give up now.

2:10 pm: I wrote him an email poem and sent it. I wonder if he'll even read it or think anything about it. *My heart cries for my beloved/ Without him I am nothing…*

2:27 pm: Message from my first love on Facebook saying I should come visit. It ended with him being sent to prison. I was devastated and cried for years. We had an amazing two weeks together a couple of years ago, but realised it was time to part ways, and we broke contact. I reply that the last ten years have been hard on us both, and that we have been through so many good times together, but the bad times will never be forgotten, and I hope he understands that the past needs to stay away from the future.

5:30 pm: Sam texts that he's heading to the gym, home at 7:30, then going to play cricket at 9 pm. I ask him if this is because he doesn't want to be around me? Partly.

6:00 pm: Sam just walked through the front door, went into our bedroom and didn't say hello.

7:15 pm: We played Wii for the last hour, he's still playing now. We didn't really speak. He said that he can't look our housemates in the face because he is so embarrassed by our show last night. He's so bothered about what everyone else thinks, but my feelings don't matter?

8:57 pm: Sam just left to play cricket. He reluctantly gave me a peck on the cheek. I tugged at his arm and said I hadn't left so he had to kiss me. He said he didn't want to yet. I'm heartbroken. I should visit my family tomorrow. I've stayed here today just to wait for him. Why is it me that always ends up in these situations? All because I slept with a guy when Sam liked me but didn't have to guts to tell me.

11:30 pm: Sam's back. He enjoyed the cricket but hadn't batted as he didn't have a cricket box. I say that he might order one on the Internet, and he spent the next hour ordering a box and some pants. Zzzzzz.

12:30 am: We lay in bed and watch *Paranormal Activity*. It was okay; he was really scared. I got to cuddle him, not because I was scared of the movie, but because I was scared of where our relationship is going.

3:00 am: We lay together in the dark and I couldn't stand the feeling that he may not want to be in bed with me, so I turned my back to him. But then he said he wanted to kiss me, he said he missed it. And we did, and we made love. I felt like I'd missed him for so long. But even though we made love, and it was really good, I still feel a little distant from him. And I asked him if he thought he'd be breaking up with me, and he said he didn't know, and asked if we could just forget everything and enjoy the moment. Did he only have sex with me because he was horny and it's been almost a week? Not because it was me and he wanted to be close to me?

FRIDAY

9:30 am: Awake because Sam's phone is ringing. He says it's his sister, but I don't know if it really was.

12:39 pm: It's Good Friday, and me and Sam have just got out of bed. He's playing Nintendo Wii. My first thought was, 'I love waking up next to him every morning.' My next thought was, 'When I get my own place like he wants, I won't get to wake up next to him every morning.' Instantly made me feel sad.

1:00 pm: We've cuddled in bed and both decided we'll go to the gym together, something we don't do usually. I don't want to spoil it.

3:00 pm: Readying to go to my parents' house for the holiday. My parents don't know I'm living with Sam and would disapprove. I come from a traditional Asian family and so does Sam. His family is a lot more traditional than mine, so I have asked him to not tell them about me yet. If and when he decides that he wishes to settle down with me then he should tell them. I've wanted my sister to meet Sam, but something always goes wrong. Usually a fight with him and we cancel our plans. Anyway, when I got back from the shower he was surprised I'm about to leave, and pulled me back to bed. Shows how much attention he pays.

3:57 pm: We got intimate. We ended up just having oral sex, but it was amazing. I covered his penis with chocolate and licked it all off. It's very new to me as I've never really tried giving head to anyone before, but with Sam I want to please him and I think I did!

4:20 pm: Showering again. Something he just did really annoyed me. He's been sporting a really strange moustache, despite my asking him to get rid of it. But now that he's going to see his family, he can shave? I got upset and started crying. He carried on getting ready and sang, ignoring me. Something's changed. I know he just sees this relationship as temporary now, as opposed to before when he made me believe we'd be together forever.

5:30 pm: We had some food just now and went our separate ways.

6:49 pm: At home with my sisters. I weighed myself, I've lost five pounds. I have been on a no-food diet after Sam has been pestering me to go to the gym.

10:00 pm: I rang him a little while ago; he was playing with his baby nephew. Cute! I told him we should stay home until Monday. If he wants to spend time with his family, I should encourage him.

SATURDAY

1:40 pm: Woke up late. Sam sent me a text last night after I'd fallen asleep. Says he's going back to Manchester tonight and hopes I can make it back too. So I will. I feel confused about our relationship.

7:42 pm: Asked Sam if he knew what time he would be back and he sent me a quick message saying he has no idea. I need to know what I'm doing and be planned, but with him in my life I can't do that.

10:43 pm: I'm in Manchester now, sat here waiting for Sam. He's not answering his calls. He's the one who said to come back to Manchester, and now he's not even here. Oh, I'm so tired of all of this!

12:19 am: Sam got home half an hour ago. He's surprised me by saying that we're going to Chester for the next two days, as he knows I want to get away. Soooo sweet. I love my man for actually listening! I just want to cuddle him. I'm very happy right now. ☺

—⁓—

the sunny young marketer too distracted by her wide and varied sex life to do any work

23, FEMALE, EAST SUSSEX

SATURDAY

9:02 am: Have just woken up, and Liz's already out of bed. This is unusual for the weekend! I was hoping for some sex last night – a day without intimacy feels like it's lacking – but I zonked out before she could join me.

10:15 am: Had a nice bath together, gently touching each other in a warm bubble bath. I love that our sex life can be so varied.

11:42 am: Sun on my skin, soft hand in mine and sweet lips on my own let me know that I'm right where I belong: in a year-long relationship with a beautiful older woman. I've never clicked with anyone in this way – a revelation!

2:30 pm: Out shopping with Liz, and just bought a glass dildo for the harness, and a double-ended dildo. Very excited about using them. In her previous relationship, she wasn't able to do as much fucking as she'd have liked ('typical' butch/femme roles), but we're both on the 'femme' side of things, and we're pretty balanced. We both feel able to be more dominant if the mood strikes, though I'm more turned on if she's the one being dominant/rough.

4:30 pm: Having such a happy day wandering around the city in the sunshine, hand-in-hand.

5:15 pm: A stranger just invited us out on a boat with a group of people tomorrow. Have a funny feeling the guy liked Liz, and hadn't twigged about us being a couple – we don't exactly look like lesbians! I want to go, it'll be an adventure and we'll maybe meet some nice people. Liz is willing but wary – does this difference in attitude show our age gap?

7:00 pm: I'm so horny, have been all day. I desire Liz constantly. She's out walking the dog.

1:13 am: Liz and I just finished snuggling on the sofa, talking about jealousy. It makes me feel loved to know that she gets jealous sometimes. And even more loved to know she trusts me. We're crashing now. Not much of our sex happens at bedtime. I think that's a big mistake that couples make.

SUNDAY

8:28 am: I'm disappointed because we're not going out on the boat after all. Trying not to accidentally ham it up. Liz says she didn't warm to the guy, and doesn't want to leave the dog. I'm feeling miffed because I often feel restricted by her dog.

8:45 am: Overcome the niggle by suggesting we go out on a picnic in the sun *with* the dog.

2:05 pm: No picnic. Instead lounging around in bed, and enjoying the sunshine. I feel so happy being able to talk to my partner about anything – she's always up for a good debate and cares about my opinion.

3:00 pm: Liz is out walking the dog, and I am pretty much gagging for it now. Two days feels like a long time. We have sex about five days out of seven, and often once earlier in the day, and later too.

8:37 pm: Just walked into the bathroom and she was on the toilet – just that glimpse of her flesh is enough to take my thoughts to sexual things! She laughed at me giving her a pervy look.

10:13 pm: Phooo. The last couple of hours has more than made up for the weekend. She went all dom on me, tying me to the bed by my wrists, and teasing me before fucking me. She put our black rubber gag with a dildo on it on my face, and sat on my face – what a view! She is so sexy and uninhibited. Then we used the new double-ender together! She ended it by using it on me while laying between my legs, using her tongue and chin on my clit. Once I'd orgasmed, she held me and touched me.

10:45 pm: Just got carried away again: she worked her fingers firmly on my G-spot while deep, intense waves washed over my whole body for a while. Now, cuddles!

11:53 pm: Liz is having a cup of tea, so I snuck a moment with the Hitachi Magic Wand while enjoying my recent default masturbation fantasy: being double penetrated, trying to 'feel' my ass being fucked. I've had a butt-plug in while she's fucked me, and Liz fucked me in the ass a few days ago. My orgasms are so strong during anal. I'm quite a difficult sub, and won't submit without a struggle first – which is lucky, because she's much older and stronger, so the only way out of a situation is to use the safe word.

11:54 pm: For now: FOOD! I am so hungry.

MONDAY

10:24 am: Lovely to begin Monday morning with cuddles in bed.

11:00 am: The plumber came around to fix some taps, and I purposely left a couple of dildos visible in the window because Liz said not to. Hoping I'll be punished later.

1:04 pm: Just had a bath with Liz, and sex while we were in the bath. I started working a finger gently into her ass, then my thumb in her pussy, and it seemed to be the right thing for the moment. Knowing that I can give her pleasure so easily makes me feel quite confident.

1:06 pm: I love working from home. I do marketing. She's gone to get us a coffee.

3:39 pm: She's gone to the bank and I'm lounging in front of the living room window enjoying the warm breeze. Life is good.

4:07 pm: Wondering about our sex life: Are we more kinky than most? Pretty much anything is fair game (excluding pee/scat/blood). Except I'm not as into spanking as she is, and she doesn't like being choked the way I do.

4:25 pm: She looks so sexy in a vest. I just snuck up behind her while washing up, and slid my head over her bum and down between her thighs. She asked me to remind her to get some dishcloths. Guess her mind isn't on sex right now.

4:28 pm: Put the glass dildo in the freezer – seems like the right weather for it.

7:26 pm: Well, any plans to get some work done went out the window. Munching on grapes after a long fuck. Feel all wobbly. She took me through to the living room, kissing me. She removed my trousers and pushed me on the sofa as I pretended to resist, then pushed my face into her slick, wet cunt and worked two fingers into me. And then another into my ass. I wasn't prepared for it and cried out. She told me to shut up, and that she'd do as she liked. Then she grabbed my throat and kissed me. I love it when she does that. Nothing turns me on as quickly or effectively as her hand on my neck/throat.

7:28 pm: Her cunt does this amazing thing when she's all turned on, it kind of opens up. It's pretty easy to make her squirt, and then she's gushing all over my hand. When she's really wet, I know I can fit my whole hand in there. This is such an intimate, and intense thing to do that it can be quite overwhelming. She has really strong orgasms from it, so I don't hesitate. She caused a puddle on the sofa (leather, thank God!). I brought her down gently, holding my hand firmly over her pussy as we kissed.

7:30 pm: Worried a little about work–life, we work together and I'm very distracted and unmotivated. We can easily lose a couple of hours once things get started. We're absolutely useless at quickies.

9:34 pm: Ahhh, feeling so loved-up. We've been snuggling on the sofa kissing, cuddling and talking. In my last relationship I told lies to prevent arguments. Wasn't unfaithful, but I felt I had to lie to make life easier on myself.

10:15 pm: Kissing turned to rolling around, turned to breast-rubbing and tribbing. I came for the first time today, even though we were fully clothed. Lesbians have all the fun – so many different ways to enjoy each other. Never thought I'd be able to talk about everything with someone.

11:49 pm: Liz's mum called while she was out with the dog. Liz got this goofy look on her face when she came back in – she thinks our chatting is sweet. So tired, just cuddles tonight I think.

1:22 am: Oops, just had more sex! I went down on her, then finger-fucked her. Two orgasms for her. Now she's going to give me a back rub while I drift off.

1:24 am: Liz: 'I wish I could keep a diary, so I can write about how amazing you've made me feel today.'

TUESDAY

12:00 pm: Liz let me sleep in. She hadn't showered yet, so when she came to wake me, I pulled her onto the bed and we kissed and cuddled for a while. Her skin is so soft and smooth and we got carried away. She pulled me to the edge of the bed and kissed down my body, until she was kneeling in front of me, lips on mine, tongue exploring my pussy softly, searchingly – like it was the first time… until the doorbell went. Postman. Bastard!

1:47 pm: Feeling a bit down about work. I am in such a rut of ineffectiveness. Where's my mojo? I used to be a go-getter.

2:01 pm: Just finished a talk with Liz about making sure that her art is a priority. I think she appreciated me bringing it up.

2:05 pm: Clit feeling sensitive and cunt a bit swollen. Don't think there will be any sex today.

8:22 pm: We just had a bath together. No sex, but we talked about the fantasies we masturbate to. I told her my fantasy of being tied down and used by several men at once. She said she has the same fantasy, but for her it's about being irresistible and desired; for me it's about being dirty, used and a slut. I'm about as far from a slut as you could be in reality, but the idea of just being fuck-meat really gets me going. The man thing has more to do with dominance.

8:30 pm: Talking about rape fantasies. Liz has acted them out on me before: the element of surprise is key, so we talk about the idea beforehand, and agree that anything is fair game. Last time she just 'attacked' me one day when I came in the door. She overpowered me and was serious enough about it that it was frightening, but I trust her, and know that I can always get out of it by using the safe word. She used my face, my arse for her pleasure, fucked my throat with a strap-on, pinned me down and fucked my cunt, my arse – just didn't let up on me until she was done! It was great, high-energy sex, and I really got off on knowing I was just a piece of fuck-meat for as long as she wanted.

9:54 pm: My ex just called up to chat. He gave me some much-needed ear-bashing about my lack of professional motivation.

9:56 pm: He's become a great friend to me. I assumed I was straight for years, despite never getting wet with a man, avoiding blow jobs and envisioning Angelina Jolie's tongue on me, not his. (Previously, I could go for months without even masturbating.) After five years, he bought me flowers and sat me down to talk about how it was clear that my heart wasn't in it in the same way that his was. We care so much about each other, though I think he's having trouble moving on.

10:30 pm: Liz just said goodnight to my ex (I love that they can do that), and gave me a back rub. We'll fall asleep cuddling.

WEDNESDAY

11:09 am: I just had the best sex of my life. I awoke turned on, put on the thigh harness and used the dildo on her for a while then asked her to fuck me in the ass. It felt so good having her on top of me, using me. She came from the pressure of the dildo base rubbing against her clit. Then as soon as I touched the Hitachi to my clit I came, hard – no build-up – just a strong, intense orgasm.

11:15 am: It's been a surprise to us both how something as scary-seeming as ass-sex could be *so* good once you get past that fear. I'd tried before and found it unbearably painful, until we read a blog about it. It didn't hurt at all because I was so turned on. It has hurt a bit since, on occasion, to begin with, but only initially. I'm a bit sore now, though.

11:17 am: Although we tried to act out the scene from *Last Tango in Paris* once, and let me tell you: *butter burns!*

2:13 pm: Liz and I are having a serious work talk: whether it's what I really want to be doing, that it's okay to change my mind if it's not. Worried.

8:32 pm: Feel as though we can sort this work thing. I think perhaps I need to get office space, so we simply don't have the opportunity to be all over each other during the day.

8:49 pm: Liz is letting me wax her bikini line – a small triangle, nothing on the labia. She gets off on the pain a bit, and the touching. It doesn't work the other way around, though – I hate it.

11:51 pm: We were just getting ready for bed, and she needed to go to the toilet, so did I. We were goofing around and giggling I climbed on her lap as she sat on the toilet. I tried to aim between her legs. Suffice to say my aim isn't all that. Oops. For some reason it cracked us up.

12:30 am: Just hanging out and chatting tonight. Eyes are sleepy. Probably no more sex today.

THURSDAY

11:40 am: Just took five minutes to take myself off to the bedroom by myself. Laying back down on our bed, imagining a completely impossible scenario: her beneath me, lifting, and pulling open my arse cheeks while screwing me in the arse, while she also touches my breasts and clit. As I said, impossible, but works well for a private moment.

—m—

the blissful skier in a dull long-distance relationship

22, MALE, LONDON

THURSDAY

9:59 am: Coffee in hand, just sent a text to the girlfriend. She's in Spain for the winter. I'm in the city sitting at a desk and she's skiing. I'm happy for her, jealous of her and missing her a lot.

3:31 pm: Chatting to the girlfriend on Skype. I always feel turned on when we Skype, even at work. Can't wait till Sunday when I see her. It's been three weeks.

3:34 pm: The long-distance thing kinda sucks. I want her right now.

4:30 pm: Just saw an attractive lady walking down the street. I often imagine having sex with other women. I think, 'Oh yeah, she's hot/fit/nice, I definitely would.' I am completely confident that I would never be unfaithful; they are just thoughts and not actions. Also the majority of my sexual thoughts are about the girlfriend.

7:28 pm: I've been with the girlfriend for two and bit years (and yes, I do know the specific length of time). This relationship feels different. Time literally flies, and I am very relaxed and feel more comfortable than ever before. We're currently apart but we chat every day and I feel we are very close. I am in love with her and I think about her all the time.

10:39 pm: Having a relaxing evening in, alone. The girlfriend has gone out for a meal with her colleagues. Wish she was here. Only three days to go.

11:05 pm: Thinking about how we met: we were both skiing one day in the first term of uni. She actually broke her arm that day, so I didn't see her again for a week. Then five months later we were both on a ski trip. I was currently seeing a girl, but I wasn't really into her. One night I bought a round of ten vodka shots, and she did very well in deflecting six of them toward me. Then she bought another ten, repeat. So anyway, we kissed. The rest of the holiday was awkward. Back at uni, we kissed again and I broke up with my ex. That was two years ago.

11:14 pm: A little five-on-one* before bed, with a little assistance from the good old-fashioned Internet. This is the part of the day when I really miss a kiss and a cuddle and so on.

11:30 pm: A very early night. Expecting a phone call goodnight soon, so will stay awake for a little bit. Relaxed, ready for sleep.

FRIDAY

10:15 am: Just woke up. Day off today. Feeling pretty turned on for some reason, thinking about the girlfriend, going to masturbate before breakfast.

1:15 pm: Skype video chatting with a friend from uni in the Caribbean. We are very good non-sexual friends, but she has great boobs. I'm looking at them quite a bit during the chat. Is that bad? I am listening to everything she says.

---

* Masturbation.

4:50 pm: Just cleaned my room, ready for the girlfriend. Got her a very nice Divine Easter egg. It's fair trade, so she'll like it. Can't wait till she gets here. Feel like I should do something productive, but will probably just have another cup of tea.

7:00 pm: Saw my ex at dinner. She was crazy for sex but she wasn't for me, though I met her parents and everything.

9:54 pm: Got a mild case of man flu (a very mild cold), so I'm not really on it.

11:39 pm: Girlfriend sounds sleepy and happy. She went out for a drink with co-workers. I feel like most people would feel jealous but I feel nothing but trust. It's a great feeling.

11:51 pm: Being alone is a great excuse to stay up and watch crappy television. 'Just go to bed.' 'Why?' The battle goes on.

11:53 pm: Two days till I have someone to cuddle.

SATURDAY

10:00 am: The mild man flu is making my eyes water.

11:44 am: Introducing Laura. She's my flatmate. She's also a lesbian. Guys get quite excited about lesbians, but I personally find it a real turn-off. If you're with a girl, you want her to be thinking about *you*. Not another girl. Laura's cool, though.

11:49 am: Just texted the girlfriend that I'm going to see her tomorrow. I'm meeting her at the airport, can't wait. She wants us to do a ski season after uni, and I do too, but I also feel like I should get a job.

12:01 pm: Heading out to a female break-dancing show, of all things.

5:25 pm: Break-dancing was pretty good. Not a massive fan of the girls with really baggy clothes. Very talented people, but they look like they're wearing their dads' trousers.

6:00 pm: Laura's friends all chatting about who slept with who the night before. I like going out, but I also like going home with a great person.

10:12 pm: Forgot to add that my parents are also coming to visit tomorrow. They're staying in a hotel. I was brought up a Christian, and at home the girlfriend isn't allowed to sleep in my room, which is rubbish. Here, we stay together. I know Mum isn't keen on the idea. I don't think Dad has an opinion.

11:37 pm: Just spoke to the girlfriend on the phone, she's excited. Can't wait till tomorrow. I like that she's independent. I had several relationships where the girl was like a lap dog and I just got bored.

11:38 pm: I'm going to masturbate right now, that will help me sleep.

SUNDAY

8:35 am: Didn't sleep very well last night because I was excited. This is our longest time apart.

10:07 am: Off to the train station to meet the girlfriend. Butterflies in the stomach, it feels like a first date.

11:30 am: Waiting in the arrivals area, just sipping a coffee. Only thinking about one thing: a big kiss and cuddle with the girlfriend.

2:35 pm: Sitting here like a restless puppy. She's showering.

3:35 pm: Damn. My flatmates are here and we're meeting my parents soon, so we'll have to wait for sex.

4:45 pm: We didn't wait, and it was awesome. Waiting really builds up a lot of passion and expectation, but it was everything I was waiting for. Ahhh, very relaxed now.

7:46 pm: Out with the parents now. The girlfriend is really relaxed and very comfortable chatting with the parents. My mum is always interested but I'm typically guarded when talking about our relationship, as a son should be!

11:30 pm: My girlfriend is really hot. She loves it when I'm on top and she likes it slow. I like it when she's on top. So we took turns and made each other happy.

MONDAY

9:52 am: It's amazing how much one misses the small things. This morning we just lay there and cuddled and chatted.

11:39 am: Met the parents for breakfast at their hotel. Off to the Design Museum for a day with the girlfriend and parents.

2:19 pm: First time for the parents in Pizza Express. We aren't big displayers of public affection, holding hands is standard, though.

6:04 pm: Cuddling while on our laptops.

11:29 pm: Back home after everyone had fun at a meal out. Looking forward to a bit of time for the girlfriend and I to spend together. Hopefully she won't be too tired for some fun.

12:15 am: She is too tired for some fun. You know, I really fancy her and she's really hot and I of course love having sex with her, but it is part of the relationship, not the focus.

—⁓—

the kinky bride marrying a much younger man

53, FEMALE, LONDON

SATURDAY

8:30 am: Woke up at a friend's house wondering where my fiancé's stag night ended up. The last text I got from Harry, at midnight, noted that there was no sign of the stripper. I don't have to worry that he's tied up in women's clothing in the back of a van in Calais. He doesn't drink or do drugs, half his stags were women and his best man is Mr Sensible. He's just never been into wild nights. Not like his fiancée used to be.

8:34 am: I'm getting married in four weeks. Emotionally, I am the happiest and most stable I have ever been in my life, and I'm 53 so I should know. My fiancé, Harry, who is over 20 years younger than me, is the kindest, sweetest, loveliest man I've ever met and he adores me. I've lucked out, and it is proof that miracles exist.

10:30 am: I'm guessing the groom-to-be and his brother are sleeping. I feel slight anxiety, but deep down know that nothing is wrong.

11:30 am: Panic over. He's just woken up. A big smile creeps across my face. Just thinking about him makes me feel idiotically happy.

12:00 pm: Back home now, and a quick hug with my intended, before rushing out to shop for wedding lingerie. I've spent so much money that it doesn't seem profligate to buy two sets of expensive scanties. I am a bridal cliché, but I don't care. I'm a lady of a certain age who never thought she would get married.

2:30 pm: Sorely tempted by the waterproof purple handbag-sized vibrators in Myla. The sales girl asks if there's anything else I'd like, and I imagine her saying, 'Something for the weekend, madam?'

3:00 pm: Another store, another set of unforgiving mirrors. Flesh seems to have gathered in folds around my slightly sagging 36D bosoms while I wasn't looking. My cup runneth over. I sometimes wonder what Harry sees in me. It's a miracle that I've found a young man who loves older women in all their fleshy glory. I think he's a perv. Correction. I know he's a perv.

6:00 pm: Home showing Harry my bags. He's not sure whether it's bad luck to show the groom. He pats his knee, which is my signal to sit on his lap. We grin at each other inanely and kiss. We can be very silly and childlike.

6:02 pm: Some people still refer to my future husband as a 'toy boy', which annoys me. I don't notice the age difference at all now and neither do most of my friends and family. Toy boys are for cougars.

6:30 pm: Sitting a few yards from Harry, answering an email from him, which reads, *Dear Whores R Us. What is the whore situation this evening? I'm in particular need after my stag night.* I reply: *Dear Staggerer. We have a shortage of whores this evening. One may be available at around 7:30 but she is an old dog and will probably be quite tired. Will this do?*

6:31 pm: *Yep! Let me at her. Is she really slutty?* I reply: *Yes.*

6:32 pm: *Fair enough. She better start getting ready now. I need her at 7:30 pm.*

7:15 pm: I'm in the bathroom with my black sackful of slutwear, mostly collected during the half-year of sexual abandonment I experienced before I met Harry: stockings, nylons and fishnets; bras; bedroom heels; suspenders. Today I have decided to be Doggerella. We get into character two or three times per week, and Harry likes me to adopt what we call 'whore personas', the most popular of which is Vampirella, who always wears the black wig and red lipstick. Doggerella is a bit rough and likes to do it doggy style. Though I'm feeling pretty cream-crackered, I'm happy to get into a bit of role play.

7:30 pm: Text. *Doggerella here. Ready for a bit of ruff?*

7:35 pm: My 'client' arrives and I tell him it's 20 quid, a discount. He leaves the note on the table. He grabs my arse and my tits quite hard. He says he likes the look of me and wants me to sit on his face. He loves it, especially when I almost suffocate him. Then he orders me on to the bed on my hands and knees and takes a good look at my bottom. 'Very satisfactory,' he says. He quickly disrobes and I can see his long, hard cock in the mirror. He enters me quickly. He asks what else I do for money. 'Suck cock,' I say. He stands and I sit. It's easier that way. 'You're so good,' he says.

7:45 pm: Now he wants me to sit on his dick, facing away. I do this until my thighs ache. I'm not fit enough. Then it's back to doggy, then lying flat on my stomach with him on top, pumping the whore. He climaxes pretty quickly and tells the whore to leave by the fire exit.

8:00 pm: Doggerella goes in the bathroom and changes. I come back and ask if the whore has gone and whether he enjoyed it. 'Yes,' he says, 'she was dirty and she loved it.' We laugh.

9:00 pm: Harry quickly falls asleep and I doze. I haven't come close to orgasm, but I really don't mind. I love playing the whore, I love turning him on and I like to be fucked. And if I'm being honest I prefer to masturbate to achieve orgasm. I think women who say they don't need clitoral stimulation to orgasm are lying.

10:30 pm: It amazes me how quickly we can go from whore and john, to a pair of five-year-olds. He's just brought me my evening drink. 'Hello Mrs Goo Goo,' he says. 'Hello Mr Goo Goo,' I reply in my silly voice. We hold hands for a while and grin at each other. These are our most private selves, the ones we never show to the outside world. He's my little boy and I'm his little girl. That's where the bond is strongest and I feel totally accepted, loved and safe.

SUNDAY

8:30 am: Harry always comes into the bedroom when I stir, usually to stroke my face and tell me how lovely I am. His daily ritual is to say, 'You know, I think you are more beautiful than you were yesterday.' Which means that I am approximately 841 times more beautiful than when we first met on 16 December 2007 at 7:02 pm. He apologised for being two minutes' late. My kind of guy. I'd been intensively dating younger guys online for six months, stipulating ages 25 to 40. I was accustomed to making the first move with younger men. He found my profile and paid a fee to join up, just to send me a message. He's a man who knows what he wants and goes for it. When I first set eyes on him I felt I'd known him for years.

9:45 am: Getting hitched makes your brain hold a complete review of your love life thus far just to make sure you're doing the right thing. Harry is The One, and there isn't much competition from my past boyfriends: there was Eddie, my partner in my 20s, and Walsh, who was having a financial meltdown through our later five years together. The years before Harry were sprinkled with one-offs and unsuitables.

9:55 am: It was MySpace that changed my life. I joined to find some musician friends from the 1980s. Call me naïve, but I didn't realise how many younger men were monitoring new members to pounce. Within days I was being stalked by a 32-year-old Italian musician whose messages were breathtaking in their audacity. He turned out to be even more mischievously attractive in the flesh and we ended up having a short affair. He opened my eyes to many things, including webcams, with which I started parading myself like a porn star for the entertainment of young males on a toy-boy website. I blush now: I'd do a striptease down to stockings and suspenders, play with my breasts and even use sex toys, whatever was asked of me. It felt unreal and surreal, and I could always turn it off. Then I met the man of my dreams, shut up the Mrs Robinson shop, and the rest is history.

11:15 pm: Calling Walsh. I am training to be a career consultant and he has volunteered to be a guinea pig. He insists on paying. We still have a great connection on the mental plane, but he's less good on the emotional one.

12:45 pm: Just finished. Walsh always guarantees a highfalutin level of conversation that encompasses life and the universe. Harry provides me with the corporeal and down to earth.

3:45 pm: One of the benefits of working from home is that Harry and I can share cosy time in the afternoon. He's tired from his morning work, so I bring him a cup of tea and two chocolate biscuits and tell him to have a lie down.

6:00 pm: He has a headache so I soothe his aching brow with one of my signature head massages, performed with his head on my belly. It doesn't lead to sex this time, but it often does.

6:15 pm: Intrigued by a newspaper photo of Edward VII's *siege d'amour*, an elaborate piece of furniture that allowed him to have sex with two prostitutes. No one seems able to venture how exactly it was used.

6:18 pm: The chair provides a masturbation fantasy: I am a voluptuous corseted trollop in *fin de siècle* Paris, the best whore in the house. Only the highest bidder secures my services. I'm taken on a plush velvet chaise lounge by a fat aristocrat. That does it for me, in less than two minutes, while Harry plays Nirvana in the other room.

9:30 pm: Harry is putting together the wedding playlist while I type. Even though we live in a small space, we often go into our own worlds during the evening.

MONDAY

1:15 pm: Just finished my homeopath session, which often feels like therapy. There are a couple of more letting-go things I need to do before the wedding, including making peace with a man I had a fucked-up relationship with before I met Harry. Set a date for a drink with him.

1:45 pm: Meet Harry for lunch. He says he's hoping to employ his brother. 'You can't afford it,' I say. He looks at me witheringly. 'You've been wrong about the last three things you said "can't" about.' He's not cross, just firm. I'm being pragmatic, and it's unnecessary because Harry is focused and has achieved all his business goals.

6:00 pm: Harry's tired. I give him a back massage. I love looking after him. I suppose it's my suppressed maternal instinct coming out. I never wanted children, but caring for Harry feels like mothering sometimes.

6:30 pm: Looking at a photo of myself, alarmed. I looked sort of… pouchy. Harry thinks I look lovely even with bed-head. I've always thought I have an attractive face, and certainly a distinctive nose, but never beautiful. I've certainly never relied on my looks to attract men. I believed I wasn't attractive *au naturel*, so I vamped it up. So glad that's over.

8:30 pm: Cooking sausage pasta. Before I met Harry I didn't turn on the oven for a year. Now I cook all our food. I enjoy it, because it's all part of looking after him and making him happy.

11:15 pm: Thought there was a good chance of romping this evening but we've both been doing our own things and now I'm falling asleep. Might get a visit from the midnight raider, though.

12:10 am: Sure enough. We're reading in bed, when he starts toying with his cock. 'What's that called?' I tease as it hardens. 'His name is George,' he replies. 'No, that's not his name. It's Fanny Ferret, and he requires your attention.' So I take to sucking the hard pink lollipop and, when I'm satisfied with that, mount it as he looks admiringly at my arse in the mirror, and then snuffles in between my breasts. This continues in an entirely pleasurably way as he progresses to teasing my 'naughty nipples.' We complete the process with what we call an 'arse ride', me on hands and knees and him taking up the rear. It doesn't take him long to spurt and, as usual, he falls asleep.

1:00 am: It's hard for me to get to sleep straight after sex, so I put on my iPod and imagine I am at an upmarket swingers' party watching a nubile young woman being taken from behind over a snooker table. I climax, and have to contain the physical jerking in case Harry wakes up and wonders what's going on. I relish my secret pleasure.

TUESDAY

8:30 am: Awake to smiling Harry singing an Elvis song about how pretty his girl is in the morning. He does this regularly, like a reverse lullaby.

8:33 am: Harry has promised to take my anal virginity on the wedding night. It's only happened once before, years ago when I was drunk and didn't want it. He assures me that this time will be completely different. I'm still not convinced, but my niece is a big fan of anal and has encouraged me.

9:00 am: Sexual nostalgia. Among the many adventures over the years: bondage and domination, submission, a heavy indulgence in leather and latex, exploring the female form, a threesome with a girl pal and our gay best friend, romping with a rent boy, a variety of toys and strap-ons and a string of much younger men. In the end, it was all so exhausting and it never made me happy, because I thought the real me wasn't enough. If I'd had then what I have now (a loving relationship within which I can play any game I fancy), I don't think I would have gone down all those erotic culs-de-sac.

9:05 am: Harry doesn't know everything about my past life, but that was then and this is now. He occasionally asks, but it seems to turn him on. I told him about occasional sexts from a male friend, and he wondered if I might consider a threesome. That's my boy…

10:00 am: Harry's on his way out. He pats my 'lovely, soft' bottom and kisses my nose. 'That's a lovely little nose,' he says before putting on his headphones. He promises that when the registrar says, 'You may kiss the bride,' he will kiss my nose first. It will look slightly absurd in the wedding photos.

3:30 pm: My 83-year-old mother calls. She is taking her role as mother of the bride very seriously, especially as she's had to wait so long.

4:00 pm: Just remembered that I forgot to buy tea bags, so I text Harry. He is not impressed. *You're looking at a spanked bottom later.* My limbs will be tied to each corner of the bed and his hand will show no mercy…

7:45 pm: I shouldn't have told Harry there was a spider on the stairs. I am Chief Spider Catcher. 'What do you think Mr Spider is going to do to you?' I ask. 'Rush up the stairs like a miniature suicide bomber?'

10:45 pm: It's fair to say that our sex life has suffered this week due to Harry's hours on the wedding playlist. But every night before we go to sleep we lie facing each other and gaze adoringly into each other's eyes. I wonder if we will be doing this in five, 10, 20 years' time? I hope so.

WEDNESDAY

9:30 am: I come out of the shower, hair dripping, to find Harry lurking near the bedroom door. 'I thought it might be time for your spanking.' He lifts up my dressing gown, kneads my buttock and kneels me on the bed. After a few slaps and squeals, he lets me go. 'You have another punishment. You're a bad girl and you're going to take a big fat cock.' I adopt the 'whore position', on hands and knees with back arched, and he enters me. In the mirror I can see my breasts. 'Take your punishment, bad girl.' In three minutes he is in a gasping heap on the bed and I'm blowing my hair dry. 'Have you missed your train?' 'No, I'm getting the 9:55,' he says. 'It was all scheduled.' Now that's what I call a morning quickie. Yum.

9:45 am: We both agree it is scary that two five-year-olds are being allowed to do such a grown-up thing as getting married. Yikes.

2:30 pm: Before I met Harry I was a gym bunny, slogging away four times a week. Then the relationship set in, and I preferred to stay in with a hot chocolate, a biscuit and a hot young stud, and became progressively more pillowy which he, a fan of flesh, loves. So I have absolutely no incentive from him to tone up and trim down. Bingo wings. He would kiss every millimetre.

6:30 pm: Harry meets me at the station and says he wants to buy me dinner. We go to one of our favourite local restaurants and even though I feel a bit zoned-out, we have a lovely time and he calms me down even more.

10:45 pm: Harry's best man has just left after going over arrangements. The wedding is beginning to feel quite close and real now. I'm happy to see him, happy to be marrying him, happy to be happy.

—⧢—

the young teacher who'd like more time, sex and a ring from her childhood sweetheart

21, FEMALE, CENTRAL BELT SCOTLAND

TUESDAY

8:05 am: Alarm went off at 7:15 this morning – and then on and off for the next 45 minutes while we were kissing and groping. It was awesome, and made me feel very wanted. I hope he is in the same mood when he gets home.

10:00 am: Just had a cracking self-induced orgasm. I was imagining giving a lap dance to that hot footballer guy who came into school to do fitness work with the kids.

10:16 am: I am a bit bored waiting for the delivery men to call.

12:30 pm: Making lunch, talking on the phone with my mum about Mark. I feel so happy that I have already found someone so amazing at a young age. I feel like we will be together forever.

4:30 pm: Mark popped home briefly to pick up his uniform for work He was lovey-dovey, and said that he will be thinking of me until he gets home. I'm going to shower and shave all necessary areas for a night of fun.

7:00 pm: Obsessing about the future. I love Mark with all my heart. Sometimes I worry that he is too busy and that I am holding him back. I find it hard to live in the moment because I obsess about the future – children, houses, marriage, etc.

10:50 pm: Mark is in the bedroom watching WWE. Feel a wee bit rejected. Thought he would come home and jump into bed. Out of the mood.

WEDNESDAY

10:09 am: Went to the bedroom where Mark is sleeping, to tell him that I managed to get gig tickets. He was all moany, and said that I 'interrupt him whenever I want!' Well, sorry. He should be up anyway – he's meant to be doing college work today. I need a few jobs done but I don't want to ask because I'll get moaned at.

11:00 am: Just asked him to give me a lift to the shops, and he downright refused to get out of bed until I'm ready! Because, 'What's the point of getting ready when I'm not ready?' AGH!

12:00 pm: Errands. Picking up parcels, going to Pets at Home to get our house bunny some food. Sunshine of my life. We are getting on well today, no silly arguments.

3:00 pm: Mark is away at a meeting for a charity, then going straight to work after until very late. He is always away doing this or that. He basically has three jobs, as well as college. I'm glad we live together, or I would be seriously annoyed.

5:00 pm: Bored, watching TV while lazing on the new settee.

7:00 pm: Masturbated. I needed to christen the new settee. I thought about a woman. I really, really, really want to be with a woman. My only regret about getting into a long-term relationship at such a young age is that unless we break up, I'll never fulfil my fantasy.

7:05 pm: I feel it's a bit unfair, really, since Mark has got to live out his fantasies. He has tied me up five or six times, which at the start it was just to indulge him, but now I love seeing him so extra turned on. We buy bondage tape because it's easier than scarves. He still wants to gag me, but I've drawn the line. Mostly because I can't breath through my nose properly.

8:00 pm: Well, I guess no sex tonight since I'm alone. We don't have sex very often, probably averages once a week. I really want more, but he says that I am never in the mood. That's not true! He just isn't that great at picking the right times. It all ends up in arguments, and then any mood that was there is gone.

THURSDAY

12:00 pm: Just got out of bed ten minutes ago after having a lovely, cuddly, long lie-in.

12:05 pm: We are going to lounge on the new settee and watch *Tomb Raider 2*.

2:00 pm: Film was pretty rubbish.

3:15 pm: We need to pop up to my mum's house with some wood, so I asked him to go and get dressed. Mark takes so bloody long to do anything! It really infuriates me sometimes.

7:36 pm: Mark's little sister just called to say her new boyfriend is flying back today. How romantic! I'm surprised though that their mum is being so relaxed about it. I mean, when we started going out she hated me because I was quiet. In my opinion it's better than being loud and vulgar like them.

10:48 pm: Mark just texted to say that he won't be home tonight. It turns out he has to stay in a B&B for a team-building activity. I'm so mad! I threw my phone down and started crying. I don't even know why. I *knew* he'd have to stay, but he kept saying no.

11:00 pm: I texted to ask where they're staying, but he hasn't replied.

FRIDAY

2:00 pm: Just got up. I feel lonely and like shit.

2:10 pm: Text from Mark: *Aaawwww don't be sad. I'll be home soon.* I know he can't help being away, but it's just my nature to be lonely!

4:44 pm: Mark is going to be away tonight too. I wish Mark were here to cheer me up. I really wanted to have sex this weekend and he's not here.

6:15 pm: To top it off my bloody vibrator ran out of batteries.

7:00 pm: I registered on one of those casual dating sites and had a wee look at girls like me: normal bisexual girls who want to experiment (i.e., not scary, butchy lesbians). Some of them were really hot. I've always liked girls but it is a purely sexual thing, I could *never* be in a relationship with one. Mark has always known, he's not bothered about it. He thinks that every girl is bisexual. We've joked about threesomes and stuff but would never really do it, I would get far too jealous.

7:08 pm: Mark and I met online, actually. We were on a public diary site, and I searched for my hometown and found a diary of someone who had that in their username. After four months of chatting we had lunch. A week later he asked me to be his girlfriend, and six years later, here I am.

9:43 pm: My mind has been wandering today to thoughts of being with a woman. I think about it all the time. I don't think it would have any long-term affect on our relationship, but I also don't think it'll ever happen. I'm going to go to bed soon although I hate being alone.

SATURDAY

11:21 am: At a dance competition that Mark is working at. He just told me that he shared rooms with Julie this weekend, because the B&B cocked up the reservations. She is just a girl from the organisation. I am fine with it. Shows that I have come a *long* way since last year when we almost broke up over my jealousy.

3:53 pm: Agh! Mark and I both have the same colour hair and wear glasses, and someone just asked if we are brother and sister. That really annoys me. Happens a lot.

3:55 pm: Double agh! I hate it when people find out that we have been together for six years, and they think it's a joke and that we'll be breaking up at some point. Yes, he's the only guy I've had sex with, so what?

7:00 pm: Spent all day at the dance competition. It was hilarious; I was really proud of him. He was around lots of other girls, and I was fine. Last summer we had a lot of arguments over masturbation, because he mentioned that he fantasised about other women. I don't mind celebrities, but thought that other real people meant that he didn't love me anymore. It caused a lot of bother. I realise now I was being an idiot.

7:08 pm: I should add that up until then, I only used to think about one celebrity in particular while masturbating (Brian Molko, yum). But now I think about people that I know sometimes and realise that it isn't a big deal.

7:15 pm: Need to get some exercise done and I will probably drag Mark to the bedroom and give him a blow job when he gets in. That'll put him in a good mood! I just really want to hear him orgasm.

11:00 pm: Mark is away to bed because he's knackered. I am so happy that he's home. Can't wait to get into bed with him and sleep all cuddled up. My favourite part is feeling his erection up against me, makes me feel good.

SUNDAY

10:00 am: Had the nicest-ever snuggle up this morning, I wish I didn't have to get out of bed! He looked so hot this morning as well. Wish I didn't have my period so I could have just jumped on him!

11:15 am: Over breakfast, Mark and I talk about initiating sex. He says that I don't let him initiate, or that whenever he does, I reject him. Which isn't true.

11:25 am: We're talking about my messed-up cycle because of the contraceptive pill I'm on and migraines. Sometimes I only have five or six days in a month where I can have sex. I will soon get the implant.

2:00 pm: Mark's sister and her boyfriend are here, being all very cute and couple-y. Mark is less keen on that stuff when there are other people around, and I wish he wasn't. If we are holding hands, he lets go, and it makes me feel like he is ashamed.

4:00 pm: Meeting my best friend in town. Lots of talk about marriage and babies and mortgages. I get annoyed sometimes because Mark doesn't have any interest in discussing things like that just now.

4:10 pm: We're talking about when Mark is going to propose to me. He will discuss it but only briefly, not at any length! He acknowledges that we will get married and he is always saying, 'our kids'. He is less keen on the whole house subject, but I have free reign there.

6:24 pm: Mark is meant to be bringing something home for tea. We haven't had a proper meal in the house together for over a month. Too busy! I hope he is up for some action of some sort tonight.

7:00 pm: Playing Wii Sports Resort together. It is really nice to actually do something together. We are both so busy that sometimes the only time we are actually together is in bed.

11:00 pm: Why can men not clean? I vacuumed and cleaned four rooms plus the cupboard. He did two lots of dishes, then had a break.

12:00am: Just sorted out a night out with the girls on Wednesday. Can't wait. Will wear my awesome purple platforms, though I have no intention of looking at others. Well, maybe a girl.

1:00 am: I just offered Mark a hand job, which he declined. I am severely puzzled. Clearly it's just because he has had a wank recently, but I can't figure out when.

1:03 am: I really just want to grab on to it, love it so much.

—⁓—

MARRIED

3

MARRIED & COMMITTED

the exceedingly diplomatic house husband who intersperses tidying with dirty Google searches

52, MALE, LONDON

TUESDAY

7:49 am: Woke an hour ago. W (wife) clattering in kitchen. Mendelssohn on radio. I wank, swiftly, fantasising of unspeakable acts with my best friend's wife. In real life she looks you directly in the eye. This is a demand for honesty. That makes the fantasy sex especially filthy.

2:00 pm: Watching one of my three children, Son #3, sailing beneath a good sun and in a cool breeze. An instructor mentions that he thinks buying boats for children is a waste when they're hopeless sailors. I agree. Am not sure that W would.

5:20 pm: How wonderful, a day free of lust or yearning. I seem to go for days obsessed by sex, and then it ceases. The yearning is the result of seeing something – someone – particularly beautiful. I am a creature of appetite.

5:56 pm: I've put on the stew, telephoned the insurance people, I've written an online review of a hotel and I am now tempted to enter 'erotic photography' into Google. Or shall I go and do some washing? Hmmm.

6:06 pm: Had a quick look for something in erotic photographs. Couldn't find much. I'd like to have had sex with all the women I have liked. I also wonder occasionally what it would be like to fellate someone but I cannot imagine a man attractive enough. Washing instead.

8:09 pm: W just back from work. We didn't kiss or touch because neither of us are inclined so to do. It is not a big deal. This is not a novel. She is tired but amused by the dog. I heat up the stew for her.

8:17 pm: W asks me how Son #3's day has been. It's been good. How has her day been? Exhausting. She is going to bed. I cannot stand the clothes she is wearing. They make her look fat. Her shoes are clumpy. She is fat. Fine, but wear appropriate clothes. She is beautiful. I do not fancy her right now. I do not say any of this, obviously.

9:00 pm: How do I rediscover W's sexual allure? My toothpick is my most intimate companion. Not quite fair, that, but lord do I need them nowadays.

WEDNESDAY

7:03 am: Woke early to get Son #3 off.

7:50 am: Grabbing a few minutes to punch in 'anal humiliation' on Google. Looking but not touching.

8:30 am: Making W a cup of tea. Just asked her how she is. 'It feels like it has already been a very long week,' she said. I said, 'Sorry.' I often don't actually *do* anything, although I think it is important for me to be around.

3:30 pm: Spending far too long fishing for porn. Pure fantasy, it takes me out of myself. The easy availability of porn – and in particular the immediate access to the moment's fantasy – diminishes my desire for W. On the other hand it keeps me honest. Would I have strayed without it? Dunno.

3:31 pm: I am married with no intention of being otherwise, but at the same time, almost obsessively desirous of the loving touch of another. I am in love with almost every woman I like.

3:32 pm: I think of W working and guilt overwhelms me. As ever, I have the nagging, nibbling, consciousness of my uselessness as a breadwinner. My children are the biggest favour I've done the world and are a continuous source to me not only of anxiety but of joy. I shall never be able to earn as W does, and my failure to earn anything is the chief obstacle to pure marital bliss. Although if I am honest, a svelte and obliging mistress in her mid-20s would be nice.

4:41 pm: I have had a fearful headache all day and a consequent sense of utter uselessness. Am going to do some washing up and start preparing supper.

8:15 pm: W in a huff, complaining that she feels responsible for the TV not working. She had a new system installed, in my view unnecessarily. I feel that actually she is responsible. Don't say anything.

10:27 pm: TV worked in the end. Watching football. W doesn't like football. No kisses for days now.

11:00 pm: Shall go and read *Brooklyn* by Colm Tóibín in the bath. The other day a masseuse said I had nice feet. I was touched. Why do I mention that now? I suppose the prospect of looking at my deteriorating bod as it reddens in the bath water.

THURSDAY

8:19 am: Woke up, got out of bed, dragged a comb across my head…

9:00 am: W lost a job during the night. She works so hard, it is heartbreaking. Still no loving touch this week, although I did pat her back this morning. Dentist today.

12:13 pm: Drove W to work. We kissed goodbye. Sweet. On to dentist.

2:00 pm: Is there something sexually interesting about having your mouth worked on and pain inflicted by two not unattractive and terrifically authoritative women? No, there isn't.

2:59 pm: Son #3 is poorly. High temp. Sleeps. W sounds fairly cheerful at work.

4:30 pm: I've written about 300 words of fiction. Have I thought about sex since the last post? Yes, but only in relation to the story I am writing. I have described that line of flesh that runs from the character's chin to breastbone, undisturbed by Adam's apple or necklace. It must, in some sense, be W's.

5:17 pm: While walking my dog, I passed a woman in her late 30s with a small child. I knew as I approached that I liked her shape. I waited for my dog and watched the woman go by, in the hope of catching sight of a well-proportioned bottom. It was. This wasn't a sexual event, though. Not really. It was simply a pleasing thing to look at, that bottom.

5:19 pm: I should add that women have generally had to make it very clear indeed that they find me sexually attractive. This was all a long time ago, by the way. I have never been unfaithful to W.

FRIDAY

7:30 am: Wanked in the bath, imagining the diary editor requiring me to strip in front of her and recount my most sordid fantasies.

8:10 am: Massaging W's neck and shoulders. Trying to stop her filling the dishwasher. W and I discuss some interior decoration. I'm happy with plain. She has Ideas. I accede to them.

8:11 am: She doesn't think I am taking the decorating process seriously.

12:00 pm: Reading in the loo, I just realised that yesterday's bottom was *callipygian*. A lovely word for a lovely thing.

12:02 pm: Eddie Izzard once described himself as a male lesbian. I quite often feel like that. I'd love to be a woman sought out by other women. I also envy the sexual power that women have.

5:11 pm: Delicious spring day warm and then cool. Can't remember thinking about sex at all: I have spent my time assembling various items, cooking, washing, tidying and reading poems. Gillian Clarke's 'Miracle on St David's Day' was especially good.

10:47 pm: W and I have enjoyed our evening sorting pictures and choosing sofas. Naturally we argued about both, which is as it should be. We may even have sex tonight, though I don't feel especially randy. Feeling fairly happy.

SATURDAY

6:45 am: Awoke with a raging hard-on. The best cure for these conditions is, of course, rampant sex. W is already up, tidying. I seek her out. I say, 'Have you never heard of the concept of a lie-in?' She simply never stops. Living with her is exhausting, let alone trying to keep up. I write this instead of returning to bed.

6:48 am: Decide to not even bother with a surreptitious wank.

6:55 am: I am stimulated by the humiliating nature of this diarying task. There is a sexual thrill in the knowledge that the editor is female. I suppose this is the kind of thrill the flasher in the raincoat gets. Makes me feel a bit sordid.

6:57 am: And in revealing intimate details, which have not been vouchsafed to anyone else, I feel as though I betray both myself and W. This is, of course, quite fun. Wickedness often is.

8:57 am: Had rampant sex! Followed by full English. Now reading about maps. God is in his heaven, etc.

3:29 pm: I go online to look up the value of some rare books, and find myself instead typing 'erect clits' into Google. Fascinating, but not stirring.

3:33 pm: The rare books turn out to be more interesting. Is this a function of age, I wonder?

8:04 pm: Very little to report, as I have had a thoroughly enjoyable day, doing errands, hanging pictures, mowing the lawn, playing table tennis, getting tipsy watching the football in the company of friends, entertaining a horde of youths in the basement and getting on very well with W.

8:30 pm: May well have sex again tonight, unless I fall asleep. My private life is about as satisfactory as I could wish. What I do not have perhaps is passion, but would I want it if it slipped in? Very possibly not. Mellowness is all.

—⁓—

the grandmother yearning for a good romp and a son-in-law who is less nude and flirty

52, FEMALE, KENT

FRIDAY

9:23 am: Morning diary! Been up for hours already – breakfast for hubby, youngest daughter and her live-in boyfriend, Adonis.

10:15 am: Just bumped into Adonis on the landing, on his way out of the shower with a hand towel draped around his lusciousness. 'Hey Ma,' with a slow smile and a twinkle in his bright blue eyes. I swear that boy deliberately flaunts himself to me!

11:45 am: Daughter Number Two just called. She's bored so she's bringing her baby round to visit. I am not bored, I have a million things to do but hey-ho.

11:49 am: I have a wonderful view of the garden, lovingly tended by my darling husband of 30 years, Sam. If only he tended me as lovingly as he does the hydrangeas! Bless him, he's sploshing happily around the pond.

11:53 am: Can see Daughter Two in back garden now, running with our Heinz 57 dog. Seems so very strange that my little girl playing happily outside, chirping to her daddy, has her own little girl in the pram.

12:11 pm: Daughter Three has just realised that everyone else is here, so is on her way. No doubt the remaining husbands and partners will fetch up just in time for lunch.

1:15 pm: Nine rounds of sandwiches later they are all beginning to disperse. This house is the family meeting hall and I'm High Priestess. How this happened I don't really know – obviously a result of our parenting and the lives we live, but I am grateful.

3:50 pm: Online. Someone might wonder why I choose 'Blotting Paper' for my user name. It's because that's what I am. I am an absorbent sheet of paper, used and re-used until tattooed with random ghostly imprints of other people's needy moments.

5:48 pm: Roast in the oven. Been thinking a lot about how to reassert myself. After so many years of being a shadow, pillow, buffer, even I don't actually know who I am. I am certainly not the pretty girl in the wedding photo. Nor am I the self-effacing woman with all the grandkids always milling around. Rebellion is churning in the pit of my stomach. I want to wear the coloured hippy dresses and have sex in the fields like we used to.

10:29 pm: Everyone in bed, including Sam. He seems so accepting of the way things are. Maybe he is right, maybe platonic, respectful friendship is okay, and I should stop fretting about what we are missing and be grateful.

1:36 am: I've been awake for a long time, just thinking about how we used to be. We would grab any opportunity to make love – on his mum's bathroom floor (real tricky, that odd-shaped floor), in the back of a car. The time we waited for his parents to go to bed and jumped on the sofa, not realising that his younger brother wasn't home. He came in just as we reached the point of no return, and stood in the door watching us. For years he called me Cita – Caught in the Act. Little shit.

SATURDAY

9:35 am: My feet haven't touched since they hit the carpet at 7 am – mad day as usual! We're going shopping.

1:00 pm: Oh my God! I can't believe what just happened. Sam and I had a full-on stand-up row. In the shopping centre! In front of everyone! We never row. We never do much of anything, really. But somehow it just blew up out of him wanting a shirt, and me trying to persuade him to try something different from the usual Ben Sherman button-down collar in a conservative shade. Shouting match, him all red in the face.

1:30 pm: I just cried all the way home. It all came blurb-blurb-blurbing out like projectile vomit, all the stuff that I have been pushing aside and pretending is not an issue for so long. It was in my head and then it was in my mouth and then it was out there! I told him how unhappy I am about our lack of any real connection, about how we live politely together with no depth. He got *angry*, very angry, and said he didn't understand me. He said he's not demonstrative, and never has been – why all of a sudden do I want hearts and flowers? I said all I wanted was to be reminded that we are both actually alive! I don't know what to do.

1:35 pm: All those wonderful memories, and I just want a little bit of it back, just a bit of excitement – but he is so set in his ways that I can't even persuade him to change his shirt colour.

2:38 pm: Life must go on, even in a crisis, so I'm hanging laundry. No wonder he doesn't seem to fancy me much so these days, when did I start wearing my mother's knickers?

10:01 pm: All very polite and frosty tonight. Going to bed because I can't take any more conversations about what's on the TV.

SUNDAY

7:14 am: Number Two has volunteered to host today's Easter get-together. So why am I up baking chocolate cake and sausage rolls?

11:17 am: My son-in-law popped out of the bathroom just now, all shower-clean and tousled and wearing a tiny pair of very tight purple underpants adorned with a leaping, snarling wild cat of some description. He's really beginning to worry me.

11:19 am: Yesterday I was in the kitchen looking very unglamorous indeed and he wandered in wearing his jeans and no shirt, came up to me as I bashed around in the Fairy Liquid. He kissed my hair and said, 'Love you.' For ages I have been putting this behaviour down to 'grateful little boy who genuinely loves his benefactor', but just lately it's making me uncomfortable. I am a granny for goodness' sake! I've got all my own teeth, but a spade's a spade, and this spade's a granny.

11:31 am: He is texting me all the time too – just jokey banter. I don't tell Sam when he texts because I know he thinks it's odd and I don't want to cause trouble. Is there a syndrome for very young men who want to shag the mother-in-law? Much as he's gorgeous, I would like him to back off a bit.

7:48 pm: Heck of a day. I'm shattered and peopled out.

MONDAY

10:35 am: Getting ready for a birthday party for a friend who raised her son by herself ever since the fuckwit she married left her pregnant and alone. Personally I hope he's languishing in a Third World jail with rats nibbling his balls. Obviously we all have our opinions.

11:00 am: Now for the outfit. The party will be a close group of girlfriends, all mates since school days. We all pretend to be philosophical about the passage of time and what it does to our tits, hair and belly, but for a special occasion we all madly diet, wax, shop and vie for who looks least their age. If you go too young they'll all raise their eyebrows. And if you miss your last roots touch-up, they'll offer you a chair.

11:56 am: Got the belly-bully-boob-booster in place. Torture that works. Only draw back is that I feel like a pork sausage. Adonis tells me that I 'look the business'. Didn't ask which business. Probably 'ageing social worker.'

12:54 pm: Sam just asked what I'm going to wear to this 'do'. I am sitting here in full regalia.

12:58 pm: The problem in a nutshell is that Sam and I have settled into a virtually sexless marriage, and he wants spice in the form of suspender belts and Roger Rabbit vibrators. I want to be romanced, caressed, cherished and *loved*. Trouble is, if I tell what I want and he does it to please me, it's not real is it? It's not from the heart and it won't work.

8:04 pm: Having a brill party. Sam is on his best behaviour. Since we argued, he's been bumbling around with a face like a miffed bulldog, putting 'if you like' and 'if that's okay with you' after every utterance.

11:21 pm: I need to sleep. Too much drinkies. Tomorrow everyone goes back to work – woop, woop. At least that cuts the blighters down by half.

TUESDAY

9:26 am: Number Two is in crisis, sobbing incoherently down the phone that she is on her way to me. My quiet day out the window.

9:33 am: The phone is still hot. Number One rang and asked if she could come round and use my computer. Which means that I get a two-year-old blessing from heaven before 10 am.

10:00 am: Got Number Two sorted out. I have always worked hard to promote an atmosphere of 'Tell me anything you need to and I will not judge.' It worked. I didn't mind my kids saying to their friends, 'Oh don't worry, my mum will sort it out.' I always stuck to my promise that I would not judge. Sometimes I would think in my head, 'Oh my God in heaven, I bore a slut!' With various offspring I have been to STD clinics, morning-after clinics, police stations and counsellors. Number Two is having side effects with the contraceptive pill, and we decided that condoms were the answer for a bit… plus the odd headache when she's not up to it.

11:33 am: Numbers One, Two and Three are all downstairs in a huge melee of girls, babies, toys and empty coffee cups. Getting shoed for a walk to the shops. Pray they don't come back. Not ever, of course, but for today.

4:12 pm: Alone at last! Just left bezzy bud who lost an old friend last night. Makes my little squabbles and irritations seem pathetic and selfish.

8:17 pm: I cannot believe how far I have come since I started this diary. Feelings that I have been turning my face from for years, and now I am able to pinpoint exactly what I want. I want him to know what he has to do without me spelling it out for him: I want him to take me in his arms and tell me that he cannot survive without me, and make love to me like I am the most precious thing in his life. I used to cry after making love, because it left me feeling like I had been blessed with a holy gift! From that, to a barren and distant friendship. We had that. Everything we need to get it back is still there, I just need to work out how to reach it.

8:30 pm: The honest truth is that I am not a sexually motivated animal. My sexual needs are dependent on emotional love. Our sex life used to be wonderful, when we were completely in love and focused totally on expressing that everywhere in our lives. He was my life, and sex was part of the expression of that completeness.

8:34 pm: I also know that the fault is mine. Babies totally changed the relationship. I only see it now with the benefit of retrospect, but the change was in me and he accepted it without question. I became totally focused on the nurturing of my children, and he became a tool to facilitate that. It sounds horribly callous and unfair: I would only have sex with him if all the children were safely asleep and for him it was probably perfunctory and certainly uninspiring. I seem to have lost that side of myself somewhere. It's not that I don't think about sex, I just seem to have lost that part of me. Along with everything else that did not say 'Mother' on the label.

WEDNESDAY

9:32 am: Friends and family often say, 'You are so lucky, you have such a wonderful relationship with all your children.' It makes me want to retort, 'Oh yes, the harder I work, the luckier I get.' The honest truth is that I have what I worked so hard to achieve: an honest, relaxed, no-holds-barred friendship with the three of them. And I chose my path to the detriment of my marriage and pretty much everything else along the way.

10:00 am: I should say that I have worked on and off all through our years together, and the only thing it really affected was my relationship with Sam (it's becoming a theme, isn't it?). Every job I did was based around the children's needs and making sure I could be home when they were home. Never once thought about how Sam and I would find time for each other.

4:30 pm: Been busy as usual all day, just got home and wanted to tell you something quickly! Sam emailed me while I was out to say he was taking me away, on our own, for the weekend! I am delighted, maybe he listened to more than I thought he had the other day?

4:36 pm: Oh, and Adonis has texted me to tell me what a beautiful woman I am today. There is definitely something weird with that boy. What to do, though?

8:57 pm: I say goodbye to this special and unique diary. It has been one of the most enlightening experiences of my life. My husband is deserving of so much more than I have given him for many years, and I give my word to myself that this will change.

—⚏—

the army wife sadly managing while her husband serves in afghanistan

28, FEMALE, HAMPSHIRE

MONDAY

7:01 am: Looking forward to reading Tom's email when I get to work this morning. Not looking forward to seeing Peter and Hannah, two work colleagues, who always ask if I'm okay. I feel embarrassed that I am okay and not crying. My granddad passed away at the weekend and I'm not crying. When I told Hannah she had tears in her eyes. Why don't I?

9:19 am: The guys at work are worried about not being able to go on holiday from the Icelandic volcanic ash cloud. That's nothing! I'm worried that Tom, my husband of six years, won't be able to come home from Afghanistan on R&R. He gets two weeks R&R in a six-month tour, including journey time, so 12 days. I can't get excited because if it is taken away, I will be gutted.

11:38 am: A co-worker just asked if I had a proper chat with Tom yesterday. I didn't really, not about Granddad. I don't want to be sad on the phone to Tom every time he phones me, which isn't that often – 30 minutes each week. He tends to phone for 15–20 minutes on the weekends, then a short call during the week. Often when he plans to phone he can't due to Operation Minimise: when someone is seriously injured or killed, all communication is minimised until next of kin are told the news.

2:52 pm: Phil has just emailed me about how lovely I look today. I think he just wants me to do a private job for him which isn't work related (!). Either way, it's nice to get some flattery today.

3:02 pm: Oh shit, now he wants to take me to lunch! I hope no one picks up my emails today. I like the attention, but I better not. Sometimes when he looks at me it's like he is mentally undressing me.

7:36 pm: Tom hasn't emailed me tonight. Most days I usually get at least one, first thing in the morning and then a few throughout the day, usually three in total. He has been in Afghanistan for 61 days and there are loads to go. We no longer have a closeness physically or emotionally. Our conversations and emails to each other are about day-to-day basic stuff (just working, going to the gym, him managing to get a bit of sunbathing in). We put on a brave face for each other and don't talk about how we really feel. We are doing what we have to, to get through it. Feel a bit sad. Guess I was hoping for a 'Are you okay and hope you sleep okay tonight.' He has no idea how crap I feel.

10:53 pm: Some nice joking comments from old friends on Facebook. I miss them. Army life has split my life into sections. It's such a huge element that the things that bother my non-army friends about their husbands don't bother me: arguing over housework, work schedules and TV channels. It makes me feel like I understand more about life and what is really important.

TUESDAY

10:40 am: Haven't really been thinking this morning. Feeling a bit down but not sure why. I'm feeling silly about being down about nothing. Hormones!

11:00 am: Emailed Tom mentioning that I feel a bit down.

11:15 am: Peter told me last week that he feels I'm depressed. I've been thinking about it ever since. I am newly resettled, and work quite far away from where I live. And I have no friends and family nearby, so no wonder.

3:11 pm: Edda commented about Phil's intentions towards me. Uncomfortable. I don't want someone else interested in me when my husband can't be here for me.

8:06 pm: Tom emailed to see if I want him to phone me, which I do. Waiting impatiently.

9:00 pm: Telling Tom that I am going to talk to the doctors about the mood-lifting pills they offered last week. Tom doesn't sound too impressed. I feel stupid! Talking to him about it means the depression will always be there at the back of both our minds. I will never be able to hide from it or pretend.

WEDNESDAY

9:30 am: A co-worker just asked how I cope with Tom being in Afghanistan. The reality is that I don't cope. I just manage to get through it. We do.

1:43 pm: During Tom's tour I'm growing flowers and veg from seed. By the time he gets home we should have loads of veg to eat. It keeps me busy, and I feel like I'm getting on with something because some days it's hard to get on with the day-to-day stuff.

3:09 pm: I'm trying to be a bit more playful today in my email to Tom, and he did the same back. I really like that, as we are always so serious all the time. I want us to have fun again.

7:59 pm: My doctor tells me I have depression, and has given me some antidepressants. I took one as soon as I got them, but by the end of the day I regretted it – for two weeks, there are a giant list of side effects to be had – and put them straight in my bedside table drawer. I want to be the 'real me' when Tom comes home. They are there if I need them on the second part of his tour. Drugs stop you feeling the real stuff. Even when it hurts bad, at least it is real! I don't believe I am depressed, just sad from feeling so lonely over ongoing periods of time.

8:06 pm: At least I feel lonely because we are apart. It would be much worse to feel lonely even when you see your husband every day!

9:12 pm: I hardly thought about anything today. I was constantly tapping my foot and trying to keep my eyes open. I'm finding it hard to see an end to all of this, if there is an end?

THURSDAY

7:22 am: My sister-in-law Jo went into labour yesterday. When I first found out she was pregnant I was happy but completely jealous, as Tom and I were trying for a baby. Then Tom got promoted and posted abroad. We had just bought our house, so we decided that I would stay behind. That was the start of my mood shift. It must've been so hard for Tom; his wife had chosen not to move with him. Then he was sent to Afghanistan.

7:23 am: Work takes us away from the people we love, but it has to be there. It makes us us. It's because I want a career that I no longer follow my husband from posting to posting. But we have been putting off having a baby as Tom is away a lot. I don't want to put it off any longer. I just want it so much.

10:56 am: I'm an aunty! I have a niece! I hope me and Tom get to be a big part of her life. I have very good memories of time with my family. I feel sad that I don't know them so well anymore. I'm interested to see how Tom's brother is with the baby. It will give me an idea of how Tom will be as a dad.

3:58 pm: Kelly, my only army wife friend at work, came over to talk. She looked tired and sad and told me that her husband might have to go to Afghanistan this year. A few months after the birth of their first baby. I feel the pain in her voice. She believes that he doesn't need to be there, as someone is already there to do the job he would do. But the army doesn't care about that. No, it doesn't. It cares about the job.

8:43 pm: Annoyed that I've missed Tom's phone call tonight. I must have been in the garden. He left a voice mail that sounded like a work-related message, not a message to a wife. He must think that I just get on with my life as normal and must be off enjoying myself. The reality is that that I am constantly waiting for him to call, and then we talk very little.

10:55 pm: Sex isn't something I have been thinking about this week. There are times when I think about it quite a lot: about experiences I've had with Tom and with previous boyfriends, or about guys I know and what it might be like with them. I don't know why I do that – I don't want to have sex with anyone else. They are just thoughts. There are not loads of opportunities with Tom, so I just make stuff up in my head when I'm doing something boring like admin at work, or quite often when I'm supposed to be listening in meetings. My mind is totally elsewhere, on sexual encounters I would like to try out. It usually brings a smile to my face and I hope no one asks me what I'm thinking about.

FRIDAY

6:43 am: There are four weekends to get through before Tom comes back on R&R. It's easier to count weekends. But weekends are the hard part. They are family time. I try to find something to do, usually involving organising the wardrobe or cupboards. I even thoroughly clean the cooker and the window frames, even the parts no one sees. I go shopping or cycling on my own. I try and enjoy my own company. Sometimes it works and sometimes it doesn't.

10:37 am: Tom has just phoned. I'm feeling pretty good after speaking to him. He had an extremely hard day yesterday in 42 degrees heat. He sounded excited about the baby. I can't wait to get my husband back!

5:04 pm: There is a festival in town tonight and co-workers have left to meet up with their partners. Even when Tom is here, I never know whether to buy tickets, as he gets sent away so fast. Some people really don't know how lucky their lives are. Sometimes I feel scared that if we did live together for a long period, we wouldn't get on.

10:52 pm: Back home. I don't enjoy socialising with couples when I'm on my own. I look away when they get all cosy. I actually hate it.

11:12 pm: I was asked recently to remember the first year of my marriage. We both enjoyed dance music and clubbing, and that's where we met, at a nightclub, when I was 18 and he was 20. I was wearing hot pants. He was a man of little words. Not very affectionate and not very chatty. For the first two and a half years, my parents kept my old bedroom, 'just in case I needed it again.' I guess they didn't think we'd last.

11:15 pm: So we married. His first posting was abroad. I gave up my job, my family and friends. We only spent a couple of months together, and he was sent to Iraq. I couldn't stop crying and stayed home in case he phoned. I had a lot of nightmares about Iraq. It made me extremely forgetful. I once locked myself out of the flat and had someone break back in, only to find the key in my pocket.

11:18 pm: Much like now, things improved when I found a job, but sleeping, eating and working was hard work. But I have been through this a few times, and each time I feel like something has been taken away from me never to come back. A piece of my personality, or maybe just a piece of me. Whatever it is I am becoming empty and numb. I love my husband, and I will put myself through this again and again as that's what I have to do in order to be married to Tom.

11:32 pm: All I need is a hug from him but I have to wait and wait. I am always thinking about him so in a way he is there with me. I know he also thinks about me.

SATURDAY

10:17 am: Hannah told me last night that I looked happier these last two days. Just over three weeks until Tom is back on R&R. I want things to go perfectly. It takes a bit of time to get used to him being home. By the time we are all loved up again, I have to take him back to the army base. Time speeds up during R&R, then slows down again when he is away. He is the only thing I want.

12:11 pm: My neighbour just helped me carry some bags of soil to the garden. It's a very hot day and he didn't have his top on. I couldn't help but have a bit of a look. He has got a very good body and very good back muscles. He reminded me of Tom. He has a great figure, but Tom doesn't walk around with his top off, unfortunately. I guess that show is just for me.

5:33 pm: There has been a hell of a lot going on in Afghanistan this week. More killed, helicopter shot down and today Tom's camp got attacked quite badly.

9:00 pm: He phoned tonight to let me know he was okay. I'll go into work next week and people will talk about the stuff they got up to at the weekend and have no idea what has been happening in Afghanistan.

10:01 pm: In my bed. I'm excited to get Tom back. We have done this quite a few times now. The first time, just having him back in my bed felt strange. I sleep in the middle of the bed when he is away, but when he is back I only have the edge. In the middle of the night he put his arm around me, and I jumped and elbowed him in the face.

10:15 pm: I'm very lucky to have found someone who I love a lot and loves me back. Some people go though a marriage for many years without that. I also still fancy him. I try not to think about sex too much because I feel frustrated that I have to wait so long to get it again. But I can't help think about what it will be like when he comes home. I know it will be like the first time we had sex. I can't wait.

4

WHEN MARRIAGE IS
MORE THAN TWO

the rampantly cheating family man

41, MALE, LONDON

WEDNESDAY

8:04 am: The usual morning train journey. Wondering if the women on the train see me as The Fat Middle-Aged Man or The Older Man with Experience. Reality says former; fantasy says latter.

9:10 am: Rachael from Outsourcing arrives. I can't work out why I find her attractive. She's a big girl and, though she doesn't have a hygiene problem, always looks like she needs her hair washed. She has a huge chest and big bum, so that could be it.

10:30am: Hour-long sales meeting with my boss. After months out of work, my self-esteem is back on top. Home dynamic has changed for the better too.

12:10 pm: Text from Janie asking me to visit her office tomorrow as her boss is away. She wants to prove that she doesn't wear knickers. I decline, so she sends me a picture to prove it.

12:15 pm: Sex at home has decreased since the kids arrived, but junk sex with others has increased. Struggling to make myself feel guilty.

2:30 pm: Two-hour meeting with a local authority is brightened by the attendance of a woman with huge breasts and a very small frame.

2:34 pm: I'm not sure an erection is appropriate in a business meeting.

5:35 pm: Just had to knock next door for my spare keys. Their new nanny is bustier than the last and spilling out of a vest. Not sure I should be masturbating over someone half my age.

9:50 pm: The toddlers are asleep and Jacqueline still at work. The weekends then tend to be rammed with things to do, so the circle of fatigue rarely gets broken. Love them all, but sometimes it's fantastic to have time on my own. Doing nothing but slobbing, but it's cool to be in total charge of the TV remote control.

THURSDAY

6:55 am: My brand of shower gel takes me back ten years to Sundays of staying in all day and Mondays of aching balls.

11:54 am: Rachael in Outsourcing has a new outfit today and her boobs look huge. The boss just finished a 90-minute debrief with her. Want to debrief her myself.

12:15 pm: Moved desks to a position where I can't see her. This is torture for a boob man.

12:30 pm: Recall that Janie's invitation is open at lunchtime as her boss is still in South Africa. My resistance is waning.

2:08 pm: Just returned from Janie. She was indeed wearing no underwear. In fact, nothing at all for most of the time I was there. Sex at lunchtime always feels naughty, but even more so when you really should be working.

3:08 pm: I am now feeling paranoid in the office that I smell like I've just licked pussy, and everyone knows. She has been threatening me with oral sex for nearly three years and it was worth the wait.

5:09 pm: Another boss meeting. At the last company do up in Milton Keynes, my boss was in the room opposite. So Krystal had to sneak in and sneak out. Krystal is a longstanding fuck buddy. She is very quiet, but has a thing for sex in public places and seeing herself having sex.

6:56 pm: Home to take the kids off the nanny. The nanny seems to paint her clothes on. I'm sure women didn't look like that when I was 21.

8:00 pm: I feel happily trapped in my life. My wife and I could live without each other, but neither of us without the kids.

FRIDAY

6:48 am: Happily squashed in the Tube next to a very sexy redhead. None of my friends share my love of ginger hair, particularly matching collar and cuffs. They think it's all a bit Freudian, as my mum and sisters are redheads. Jacqueline's hair was red when I met her. It was too late once I realised it wasn't her true colour.

3:50 pm: Rachael from Outsourcing has just asked me along to an '80s Christmas do. I'm assuming it's a general invitation, but I now can't rid my mind of the image of those huge boobs being offered to me under mistletoe.

3:51 pm: It was much easier when I was permanently field-based. There are just too many tits in this office.

5:10 pm: A co-worker commented that one can't love your partner if you're having sex with someone else. Does that mean that every time you think about sex with someone else, you don't love your partner?

And does it follow then that every time you flirt, you don't love your partner? And every time you think about sex?

5:12 pm: And what about emotions? A year back a friend of mine said she believed we were having an emotional affair. Our mutual friend thought that was even worse than physical.

9:06 pm: Jacqueline has flu. This changes everything for the weekend. Tomorrow I now have ballet lessons in the morning and football in the afternoon. The big problem is having to rely on Jac's parents to chip in. Nothing will be said, but there will be disapproval of me going to the football.

9:15 pm: The plan, I should say, is to be in this relationship for the rest of my time. Jac is the only one I have ever considered spending the rest of my life with. The fact that I have been unfaithful is no real indicator, as I've never been faithful. I can't say I won't be sleeping with other women as that would be to break a 26-year habit.

9:18 pm: I will say, though, that had I met Liza when we were 36, and not 16, we'd probably be married. We loved each other's humour, company, and we took the piss out of each other constantly. She was the wife I met 20 years too soon.

SATURDAY

9:59 am: Ballet lessons are not the ordeal I thought they might be. The place is full of yummy-mummy types.

10:05 am: As I've got older, my taste in women has aged with me. I can see why anyone would want to fuck our nanny, purely from a physical point of view, but there is something very sexy about women in their 30s and 40s. A while back I had sex with a woman of 62 and was amazed by the great shape her body was in. Yet when I was 20, I thought sex stopped at 40.

11:42 am: My daughter has her two friends over. I've got three girls under four under my feet, but it's great fun. They are very competitive at such a young age, always upping the ante in terms of who's got what and who's done what. I pity the bloke that ends up with any of them!

11:44 am: I hope they're still friends when they're older. Sexual relationships come and go, but some mates are for life.

12:50 pm: On my way to the most enduring non-family relationship of my life. A mistress who has taken precedence over every woman I have ever known. She lets me down regularly, she leaves me lost and alone for the summer months, promises so much and breaks my heart every time. She has cost me more money than I care to remember. She is West Ham United. This is true love.

4:00 pm: Ah, three hours of testosterone-fuelled stupidity, cradled in the arms of sweaty men who stink of beer – like a day at the spa.

7:27 pm: Home from the football and Jac is really not well. Her mum has been here to help. I will not be flavour of the month. Coming in with dinner and flowers increased my standing, though.

10:15 pm: Looking at a drawer, where under lock and key are saucy snaps of my ex-girlfriend and I on a beach. Is retrospective home-made porn with an ex-girlfriend grounds for divorce? Everyone expected us to get married. She gave me a Get Out of Jail Free card by starting an emotional affair with the guy she eventually married.

SUNDAY

7:08 am: Here I am with two tiny people watching cartoons at a time I used to be getting in at. My youngest is only just beginning to talk, but he has mastered 'Pink Panther'. I wouldn't swap this for anything.

7:15 am: The kids bring huge joy, but take away all free time and any chance of bedroom spontaneity. That's possibly one reason that NSA (no strings attached) sex appeals. I'm not suggesting that my kids are responsible for anything I do sexually, but the restrictions they bring certainly emphasise forbidden fruit.

11:10 am: Text from Stacia. She once told me I had 'an aesthetically pleasing cock'. I would have preferred 'huge', but I'm okay with that.

11:15 am: Mobile phones have made it quite easy to meet people for sex. Some years back, before I met Jacqueline, I was chatting to anything up to 20 different women a week. Most I never met, and even I was shocked by their readiness to send me nude pictures, to masturbate on webcams, to ask me to do the same. Women aged anything from 18 to 65.

2:29 pm: Jac is shopping, and my daughter and I are doing a puzzle. This takes me back to my own childhood. Wet Sundays are for doing sweet fuck all. None of this ridiculous middle-class pressure to do activities. The kids will do whatever we do on weekends, just because Mummy and Dadda are there. My son laughs at everything. If he wasn't so bright, I'd think I had a simpleton on my hands.

11:05 pm: Rereading an email from Jennifer. We had a fling in my second year at university. She was a swimmer with a large firm bust, red hair and auburn pubic hair. My dream woman. She was very keen and I was playing the field. It can't have been that nice for her to have been picked up and dropped whenever I wasn't horny or available. I mailed her recently to say I was sorry for messing her about, and not knowing a good thing when I saw it. At the time I wrote it, I thought it might be just a bit egotistic, but she's taken it completely differently! She thinks I'm looking to restart things. She lives four hours away with her husband and kids. Where on earth does she expect me to conduct this affair?

11:10 pm: Looking at her Facebook photos. Her obsession with avoiding being overweight means she's lost too much weight. All the curves have vanished. I really don't fancy her. It's interesting to see how she reacted to what was a completely innocent Facebook message.

11:20 pm: A girl I fancied at 15 contacted me recently. After only a few exchanges, she asked to meet me. Recently divorced. I politely declined, but it really could have been sex with someone 25 years down the line, having said little more than a few words. I think I preferred the days when there was a little more effort involved in getting someone into bed. If technology has wrecked families that might otherwise have stayed strong, then that's not good.

MONDAY

8:04 am: Jac has the day off. I'm jealous as I sit on the train to Charing Cross. Especially now that some 20-stone woman has tried to jam herself into the middle seat next to me. The fattyist in me screams, 'If you stood up or walked a bit more, you wouldn't need the fucking seat so badly!' My positive Monday morning feeling is starting to wane.

8:11 am: Seat opposite has been taken by a girl of 30 who doesn't realise that her two blouse buttons are undone. She is sleeping. Suffocation by lard doesn't seem such a problem.

11:31 am: One of the girls in the office has become very chatty in the last few days. Short and a bit dumpy, but wears a bra that makes her smallish bust look huge. We just got stuck in the small kitchen together, and she asked me if I needed to get past her. I said I just needed to wash my blueberries. She said she'd happily wash my blueberries for me. We both blushed and giggled. Slight awkward silence, magnified when I turned from the sink and accidentally touched her breast.

8:47 pm: My new scream-free parenting style has been tested to its limits. Jac compounds my anger by texting as we're talking on the way to an adults-only dinner. I stop talking mid-sentence, and it's a good ten seconds before she notices. I absolutely fucking hate that. Bury my anger for the sake of a good evening.

10:30 pm: … And that is what we had. Just the two of us falling asleep over a table in a restaurant. Bliss!

11:04 pm: The babysitter has put our daughter in our bed. With both kids asleep, we make love on the sofa. Trying not to get caught by your toddlers is worse than trying not to get caught by your parents at 16. We giggle and freeze at every creak of a floorboard. Thank Christ for stair gates.

TUESDAY

5:00 am: Up for a breakfast meeting. Catch sight of myself naked in the mirror and wish I hadn't. I am beginning to look older naked than I do with my clothes on.

5:01 am: Telling myself that I've always traded on personality. Can't say I'm unhappy with the results.

10:00 am: Call from my best friend. There isn't really anything that he doesn't know. Obviously, I wouldn't tell him I'd like to fuck his wife – though I think he'd think I was gay if I didn't find his wife attractive. I'm game for anything sexually, but I draw the line at anything that hurts anyone else, emotionally or physically.

2:30 pm: I am presenting to a woman who must be 40 and at least a couple of stone overweight, but she is so sexy. I'm not struggling to stay professional, but I am already wondering whether her breasts are large and firm, or slightly saggy because of the excess weight she is carrying.

2:47 pm: Every exchange now is sexually charged. She probably has no idea how horny she is making me, but somewhere in the back of my mind, she is sucking my erection. In reality, we are discussing the terms of her contract. I have an overwhelming urge to show her how hard she has made my cock. There are two potential outcomes: she will either be pleased to see my erection, or I will lose the deal and get arrested. I am constantly amazed how close my penis comes to winning these battles of logic.

4:25 pm: On the train. Still horny from the meeting. Browsing a photography model website. Get an alert that a new model has joined in my area. She is a size 16 with amazing tits.

4:35 pm: Just found myself masturbating in the toilet of a commuter train.

5:40 pm: A girl whose shiny leggings appear painted on just presented me with a business card for a lap-dancing venue in W1. (I'm walking down Moorgate in the City, so I must applaud their recognition of their target market.) The girl alone would be worth the cab fare, entrance and dance fee. Lap-dancing doesn't do it for me, though. The mock-conversation nonsense and fakeness annoys me – it should be a straight exchange of cash for naked flesh. Just show me your tits, take your £20 and go talk shit to another moron who'll think you fancy him.

11:17 pm: Well, I have nothing left to confess. I feel remarkably at ease that my sordid wanking, letching and extra-marital fucking have been shared with you, stranger. I think about sex constantly, I take sexual risks too often, but I love my wife and kids. I'm pretty confident that in doing so, I represent the vast majority.

—◊—

the sexy expat enjoying a long-term polyamorous marriage and a trophy girlfriend

29, FEMALE, SINGAPORE

WEDNESDAY

6:50 am: I wake up alone in a starfish pose, limbs flung towards the corners of the bed. The Husband (henceforth TH) is away on business, as he is 30 per cent of the time. People assume this is hard for me, but I like my own company and the reunions are always nice. To paraphrase Audrey Niffenegger, I'm glad when TH is gone, but I am always glad when he returns.

7:00 am: I have a wank, barely awake and solely mechanical, no fantasy. The World Service clicks on.

7:10 am: After listening to the news I make myself come again, this time thinking about Potential Trophy Girlfriend (PTG). The act is as much practical as indulgent: the extra shot of orgasm kick-starts my metabolism and I drag myself out of bed.

8:30 am: I muse on PTG in the shower. 'Trophy' because she is gorgeous and [cough] several [cough] years younger than me, and 'potential' because neither of us wants to ask much of the other. We've fucked, but I wouldn't say we *are* fucking. Each time has been a self-contained, alcohol-driven event. She's coming over tonight to learn to bake (not a euphemism). I take the liberty of shaving my legs and putting on nice underwear.

4:50 pm: Hella busy afternoon at the office, punctuated by TH emailing. He's being Mr Executive – giving speeches, going on the telly, pressing flesh – and now he's feeling small and tired and needs reassuring.

4:55 pm: TH is not 'The One', but that reassures me. Our relationship is borne of hard work rather than a thunderbolt. We have had an open relationship for six years (out of eight) and while we've always known where we'd like to be, we haven't always known if we'd get there. But for more than a year now everything has been driven by Teflon-coated gears. We are communicating better than ever, we've had loads of super-enjoyable group sex, and as a couple we seem to be forming something perhaps a little more substantial with another couple (PTG and Cute Boyfriend) – which is new and exciting territory.

10:10 pm: Baked with PTG. We accidentally-on-purpose brushed against each other, and ended up lying on the sofa together waiting for the kitchen timer to ding. And then she was gone and I was frustrated. But she went to see Cute Boyfriend – he's leaving town tomorrow so I can hardly begrudge her. Fortunately, frosting fixes most of life's ills.

10:18 pm: I've been thinking a lot lately of sex with PTG and Cute Boyfriend. This is a practical issue. I have slept with them both, and she has slept with TH, but we haven't had both boys naked in the same room at the same time. This is likely to happen, but I think it might freak out Cute Boyfriend. I keep meaning to sit down with him and ask what stepping stone would make him comfortable, or where he wants to go next, but I haven't made time for that conversation yet.

THURSDAY

7:30am: Slept like I was dead – assuming that the dead have mild work-based anxiety dreams – and woke upon a World Service package about a veiled Saudi woman taking *Arab Idol* by storm. I try to put Allah out of my head as I have my morning wank. Instead I think about TH folding me in his arms and calling me a whore as he softly commands me to come.

9:15 am: Beautiful statuesque Indian girl on the commuter train. She is wearing a sage green sari edged with burgundy and copper thread, and a burgundy choli showing a tantalising expanse of stomach. She owns the space around her. I am captivated.

4:50 pm: TH emails, forlorn that he is rushing to the toilet every half-hour. I ought to counter with something like 'Oceans might divide us, but scatologically we are as one,' (I too have gastro troubles), but work has fucked me off too much to want to make lame jokes.

6:00 pm: Thinking about sex with TH. It lurches from depressing, when we get sidelined by our jobs, to amazing when we remember that it's supposed to be fun. I often feel that our sex life lives in a box, unpacked and then swiftly repacked so we can return to asexuality. I want to receive filthy emails while I'm working, or have a hand stuffed up my top while we're alone together in a lift. But that just isn't his style.

6:05 pm: He also doesn't abandon himself to sex; he is always controlled and a bit distant from the process. He often counters with 'they do it too' (they don't, but it's bad form to bring up other fucks, so I have to let that one go), or 'It's just how I am.' I'll give him that one. He always listens carefully and tries hard to respond. This is an ongoing discussion – there are times when the sex is amazing, and I remind myself that I genuinely want to be with this guy when I'm 80, sitting next to each other in bath chairs, shooting the breeze. Can't say that about anyone else I've fucked.

10:30 pm: PTG has just left after lesson two: chocolate fudge butter cream frosting. We have a lot of fun, sticking our faces in the bowl of melted chocolate and licking cream from each other's fingers. It's all very suggestive and very silly and then we drink beer and watch comedy and swoon over Noel Fielding in *The Mighty Boosh*. I'm not brave enough to make a move, but the excitement is fun. I feel teenaged again.

10:45 pm: TH and I decided to make our relationship more open after two years of failing at monogamy. The first thing we did was write a list of rules. I think there were about 12 in all, and the gist was 'check first before doing anything more than kissing'. My difficulty recalling them is because these days our relationship is more organic. We needed the safety net of rules to get to a place where we naturally knew and respected each other's comfort zones.

10:49 pm: TH was for a long time more comfortable with me fucking other girls, so the first time I spent a weekend alone with Other Guy felt like a watershed moment. Other Guy is someone I met at uni and had an amazing no-strings six months of sex with. It was basically a crush that never wore off. But in the years that followed I didn't always relate to him in a way that was healthy with respect to TH. I realised I was feeling guilty about still loving him, and therefore acting furtively and defensively, so there were no parameters within which TH could feel comfortable. Since then Other Guy and I have shared a few naked weekends, which I'm very grateful for, especially because I knew he'd settle down with a proper girlfriend and she probably wouldn't be cool with him fucking his friends. This has since happened.

10:57 pm: There's sometimes sex while TH is travelling. I had the feeling that TH would be fine with the idea, so I asked, and the agreement shifted from 'no sex without checking each time', to one that is more fluid: 'It's fine to have sex with these people in this setting without checking first'. TH sees his business trips as a chance to cut loose and pick up young ladies. I've been thrown by this when it's happened without my expecting it, but we're now at a point where I feel fine with the idea that it may or may not happen while he's away. I think the moral is that it's okay to change the status quo in small, safe increments, but if someone does something wildly unexpected, the other person is going to feel threatened and upset.

11:02 pm: Do we talk about sex afterward? The deal is that TH doesn't really want details, but he will get full disclosure should he ask. Most of the sex with others is in a group setting, and we tend to talk about it a lot afterward. It's a turn-on. It's nice to have the connection of being in the same room fucking other people – I can look over and know straight away that TH is happy.

FRIDAY

5:00 am: Slept like a dead person until 4 am, and then slept like a wide-awake person till now. My morning wank wakes me up and warms me up, but isn't super-enjoyable.

8:30 am: TH arrives home while I'm in the shower. We kiss from opposite sides of the glass as if we're visiting in prison. Running late, so manage a quick chat, but am aware that I'm short-changing him.

9:20 am: Weird cute guy on the train. He's wearing a singlet, chequered Bermudas and leather Chucks and has shoulder-length curly hair and a goatee. Catch his eye and smile. From then on, every time I peek I catch him peeking too.

5:40 pm: My work-day emotions veer between frustrated, scared, angry, militant and jubilant. Decided that I will resign on Monday. The acceptance that I can walk out, combined with it being Friday and TH being home, has me buoyant.

9:00 pm: Arrive home for the grand TH reunion, and subject him to a 30-minute data dump on the work situation. Then I drag him to the bedroom for 20 minutes of fellatio and a quick shag. It feels good, necessary. TH definitely keeps me balanced. I'm feeling great.

10:00 pm: TH and I dance around naked to The Prodigy and tease each other. A sample of a new-ish drug, mephedrone, arrived in the post this week and we decide to try it out. I should point out, while I can still type, that the drug is currently legal but is unlikely to stay that way. Friends in the know describe it as somewhere between ecstasy and coke. When we were baby Londoners we did a lot of ecstasy as it was the cheapest form of entertainment available to us, but it's been a long time.

12:20 am: The mephedrone is clean. Not really like coke (affecting dopamine), more like MDMA (affecting serotonin), but milder than ecstasy. I come up gently without any big physical waves, and mostly feel floaty and chatty. TH and I talk and talk, about our life together and how our relationship has changed, our friends in London, how we relate to our families, books we've enjoyed recently, everything.

1:20 am: One possibility we talk about is a permanent multi-way relationship, where a third (or fourth?) party moved in with us. At this point neither of us wants that, and I suspect my life won't take that direction, but if it ever seemed viable it would certainly get plenty of consideration. This year I'd like to develop relationships with third parties that have a certain amount of emotional depth and stability, similar to that of a monogamous couple who've been dating for a short while. One poly guy I know calls this 'travelling without moving', because group or secondary relationships are not necessarily heading towards the same milestones as monogamous ones, but can still develop emotionally.

2:00 am: We have some floaty sex but I am starting to crash and getting ready for bed. Pop factoid: before ecstasy was made illegal, it was successfully used as a tool in some marriage guidance programmes.

SATURDAY

11:20 am: Ahhh, Saturday morning. No World Service, no wanking, just me and TH curled around each other.

6:30 pm: Post epic nap, I am heading to the shopping centre for a massage, a bikini wax and a hair cut. Having kids is really gonna fuck up my lazy weekends. I should mention that we've been trying for seven months. Initially I timed ovulation, but each month meant two weeks post-ovulation where I might've been pregnant, and getting my period felt like a loss. So we've gone back to the centuries-old method of fucking and waiting for nature to take its course. I have been *much* saner.

11:00 pm: Got home at ten and TH was talking to my sis on Skype. I've been missing her lovely little idiot face a lot lately. My sis knows I have an open relationship, it makes her a bit uncomfortable, but she tries hard to be accepting. I tried to come out to my mother as bi when I was about 17, and she told me that if it didn't involve her grandkids, then she didn't need to know who I was sleeping with.

11:30 pm: My 30-year-old, hotshot executive husband just informed me that he really respects Lady Gaga as an artist, and is subjecting me to a large part of Lady Gaga's canon via YouTube. I get my revenge by making him listen to Apache Indian doing a cover of The Israelites.

12:00 am: We're talking about my birthday party. Assuming I can pull it off, I will celebrate my 30th with a private orgy. Have been to a few big, sort of commercial orgies in the past and never quite vibed with the atmosphere. Then last year I went to a private orgy and had a lovely time. So I figure I should take matters into my own hands and arrange them. We shall see if it works.

12:08 am: My sex wish list: First, double penetration. This isn't a huge fantasy, but I'm certainly curious, and may get the opportunity to try it out soon. Next up is knife play. This is serious BDSM edge play. At this point Other Guy is the only person I would trust to put a blade to my skin. However, I don't think I am prepared to have the conversation where I tell TH that I want to try something hugely intimate and reasonably dangerous not with him. And finally, strap-on sex. I got one for Christmas but have yet to try it out. I have a loose agreement to try it with a girl, but every time she sees me ineptly trying to put a straw in a juice carton, she jokes that the deal is off.

12:10 am: I have a pet theory that much of the way men and women relate to each other, and hence how society is structured, comes from the psychological difference between penetrating and being penetrated. So I'm very interested to see if sex feels different emotionally when I assume the role of the man.

SUNDAY

8:40 am: Wake up hung-over. Alcohol's after-effects give me lots of booze-related mood swings. It was enough to make me stop drinking for a while, but drinking is a large part of my life. Work flits into my head (Sunday = practically Monday).

1:40 pm: Yoga, feeling much better. My dry mouth, headache and bad mood told me to skip the class, but fortunately they were overruled by experience.

6:06 pm: Spend a happy afternoon at a gay pride fundraiser. Me, TH and PTG share two bottles of champagne and get giggly and flirty, then she heads off to find Cute Boyfriend.

10:30 pm: I initiate sex with TH, but I'm only doing it because it's early still, and we didn't fuck yesterday. Once we get going my head catches up with my body, and both get quite carried away (fake it till you make it?). Everything started slow with the barest of butterfly touches. Appreciative noises guided onward. He ended up squeezing, pinching and pulling my nipples and clit – never breaking the slow pace or taking his eyes off mine. There's something about the deliberateness of that kind of intense pain that makes it incredibly hot.

11:30 pm: I think we both still have the remains of the mephedrone in our systems, making us more tactile and open to emotional connections. It was one of those fucks were our bodies started to flow into each other. It's definitely the most emotionally present I've been for sex since TH has returned. It was a complete communion – tuned into each other and blocking out everything else. When sex clicks for us, it really clicks.

MONDAY

7:40 am: Wake, World Service, wank – you know the drill. I wank while thinking about being forced to my knees and slapped round my face.

7:44 am: I'm conscious that I haven't said much about being bisexual or masochistic. Truth is, I don't think much about these things. They are deeply and completely a part of who I am, and have been since I became sexually aware at the age of 14. I have never fought or fretted about my sexual inclinations – I just enjoy them.

7:50 am: A thought on wanking in front of one's partner: I have never felt self-conscious touching myself during sex, but how I wank on my own is very different. Good old Betty Dodson's *Sex For One* helped me get past this. I mentioned to TH that a big part of my everyday life was missing, and we both agreed that we needed to masturbate more than we had been, that we were fine doing it near each other, and that it was separate from sex and we wouldn't say anything about wanting to fuck each other. Not hiding our masturbation from each other is a good thing indeed.

7:42 am: Though TH is an owl whereas I'm a lark. I get annoyed if he starts to wank just as I'm falling asleep, as the motion invariably makes me wide awake again.

7:44 am: The World Service informs me that Ricky Martin is gay. This is news? Really?

9:00 pm: Work passes in a daze.

10:00 pm: TH makes sexual overtures, but I tell him I'm too tired. We remain wrapped around each other for some time.

11:15 pm: Snuggle up to TH and fall asleep with my head on his shoulder, holding his hand. I HATE sleeping tangled up with another person, so I think this is a sign of how much the day has thrown me off my stride.

11:20 pm: We've taken some massive and rewarding leaps of faith with our open relationship. My experience is that white lies or omissions can paper over the cracks for longer in a monogamous rather than a non-monogamous relationship. Thinking about this is making me realise how completely I control my life and where it goes, and how good things are worth working hard for.

—m—

the workaholic polyamorist with a husband and a boyfriend... who are both workaholics

41, FEMALE, SURREY

WEDNESDAY

7:15 am: Alarm goes off and I roll over. The other side of the bed is woefully empty. Hubby has been working away from home during the week for the last couple of months. There's not enough cuddling and, worse still, I have to make my own coffee.

8:45 am: Caffeine levels topped up, breakfast eaten, cats fed, time for work. I run my own business, so most of my human contact during the day is over the phone, or on IM; Hubby can usually log on from his office, so we chat during the day.

10:55 am: Dropping a note to Bloke to tell him that he has a parcel here. Bloke is my boyfriend; doesn't live with us, but I usually see him once a week or so. That's been getting a little less frequent over the past few months. Both of us have been very busy, and I really wish Bloke would figure out how to stand up to his work's demands for unreasonable hours, and be able to let go when he leaves his office.

11:20 am: Ah good, Hubby's out of his morning meeting at last; exchange pleasantries. Quiet morning so it's nice to talk. Hubby has a girlfriend too – I like to say that we're in a flexible, open, long-term, supportive relationship. He's my university boyfriend, and our relationship has been open since quite a while before we got married. I'd struggle to remember the thought processes involved.

2:10 pm: Much silliness on IM, largely centring on weather differences at opposite ends of the country. Well, we were amused.

8:10 pm: Evening out in the pub with Best Girl Friend. We're talking about men. She sympathises with my lack-of-Hubby problem, though is suffering from a lack-of-sleep problem (child). My friend assures me that it is not unreasonable to want more man time with both of them, and that I have not turned into raving loon due to lack of nearby testosterone. Well, that's all right then.

11:46 pm: Just got in, about to speak to Bloke. I think if Bloke was my only partner, we'd probably have split up long since, because he's not the greatest at remembering to pay attention on a day-to-day basis. But our relationship works fine as a secondary one.

12:10 am: Spoke to Bloke. He misses me, which is good because I miss him too, not having seen him for a couple of weeks. More free time to actually *enjoy* my relationships would be nice. But that would also require Hubby and Bloke to *also* be less work-stifled. And chances of that happening? Minimal.

THURSDAY

7:15 am: Wonder if five minutes with my little battery-operated friend will wake me up.

7:20 am: Not really. But it's still an improvement on the alarm clock.

3:09 pm: Family phone calls. I don't mention my boyfriend to my family because I don't think it's their business, and I don't fancy attempting to explain the situation to them.

4:30 pm: Hubby just called to discuss a point of household logistics. Nice to hear his voice – I forget how much of our communicating we do by email or chat.

6:00 pm: Making dinner, thinking that I wish I got more opportunities to be tied up. It seems to have dropped off our collective radars in the last few years, likely because it takes *time*. I'd like more occasional bondage rather than anything dom/sub. Hubby and I find that all the dom/sub stuff doesn't work so well (for us) as such long-term partners.

9:00 pm: You know, one of the most annoying things about Hubby being away during the week is the chores. Putting the rubbish out has just taken half an hour, because we have the world's most complex recycling system. Yes, there's no one to cuddle up to, but there's also NOBODY TO EMPTY THE DAMN BINS. Weekday singletonhood sucks.

9:15 pm: On the plus side, Hubby, Bloke and I are all going out for dinner on my forthcoming birthday. It saves scheduling two meals, and we all wanted to try a particular new restaurant. Hubby and Bloke get on very well. We were all friends before Bloke and I became partners, and the same applies to Hubby's girlfriend. The dynamic between the three of us is mostly them ganging up on me and taking the mickey out of me.

9:20 pm: Now, the birthday question: will it wind up as a threesome? Threesomes have happened and were very good fun, but finding a time when all of us are available and none is tired is not easy. Sadly, threesomes are not that common.

9:21 pm: More sex would be nice in general, but that would require everyone concerned to be less busy. But I feel satisfied because I'm in two long-term relationships working well.

FRIDAY

12:20 pm: The to-do list is getting longer. My university reunion is tonight, I need to attempt to not look like I've aged 20 years. Though, everyone else will be 20 years older as well.

2:06 pm: I'm hoping that two men I've not seen in 20 years will be there: R, who I fancied no end, but who simply wasn't interested in me; and N, who might have been interested had I been willing to make a move. Unfortunately, I was too shy, and he probably wasn't *that* interested, despite one of his friends suggesting that I should just 'jump his bones' already.

2:15 pm: A mutual friend on the phone is reporting that R apparently has a fairly recently acquired wife (three years) who is horribly jealous of his time at university, and is doing her best to keep him away from people he knew then. Sad, really.

3:05 pm: Right. Have dress, have shoes, have jewellery. My looks have probably meant that I've never been the most confident going out, but they've not been much of an issue during a relationship.

3:07 pm: Might as well throw in a couple of condoms. Just in case, you understand. Yes, I generally discuss partners ahead of time with Hubby. And the question has never come up with Bloke, as I've not had any other partners since we've been together. I am his only partner, and have been since we started dating.

8:00 pm: Neither N nor R are here, so no fond reunions of that type. Still, plenty of other people to reconnect with. People mellow over 20 years.

11:00 pm: Updated Hubby. There's nothing that I get from Bloke that I *don't* get from Hubby; I just get more of what they both provide. And they're not clones, but they are reasonably similar in interests and attitudes.

SATURDAY

10:30 am: Day starts quietly, with only a mild hangover. Texted hubby to advise him of plans. He responds, *She lives!* He only got up a few minutes ago himself.

12:00 pm: Potter around the town where Hubby and I went to university. Somehow it's not quite the same without him.

1:15 pm: Quick email from the man I dated before my boyfriend. It fizzled out when he concluded that polyamory wasn't working for him, but we're still very good friends.

2:15 pm: Return home to find Hubby cleaning the bathroom. Points for that. Really significant points.

7:00 pm: Hubby volunteered to come to an event tonight that I'm not sure is going to be quite his thing. We shall see.

9:30 pm: Actually he enjoyed it, and is encouraging. Picked up a Chinese on our way home.

11:00 pm: No sex tonight. Which is fine, we're both tired. I think Bloke's existence possibly makes Hubby a bit more relaxed, because he knows that he doesn't have to be the be-all-and-end-all for me. Bloke, likewise, doesn't have to be full-time emotional support. It's sort of like a job-share.

SUNDAY

9:10 am: Hah, yes! After much swearing and hitting of refresh buttons, I have tickets to an event. Hubby is fairly relaxed about having been woken up by the sound of this. Makes up for all the times he wakes me by talking in his sleep. I'll be going with my sister, since neither Hubby nor Bloke would be interested.

12:00 pm: Hubby and I are sat at the table with several large pieces of paper and two laptops, trying to work out a schedule for the next few months. It's a good thing we share the same interests, or one of us would be really bored.

3:30 pm: Tentative schedule worked out. He's now off for a run, I'm going to the gym.

7:00 pm: *Sounds of cursing while booking upcoming trip online.*

8:00 pm: Phew, all sorted. Open a bottle of champagne in celebration. He asks if I really feel like cooking, and I absolutely don't. We order a curry.

11:00 am: A lovely shag with my Hubby.

MONDAY

5:15 am: Way too damn early. Hubby has to leave to get back to work. I vaguely mumble something in his direction that might be goodbye.

7:15 am: Wake up, check mail from bed. Email from Hubby confirms he's made it to the airport.

11:00 am: No chat this morning, as Hubby's network is on the fritz.

6:00 pm: Bloke will be round for the evening later on. On chat, Hubby and I are discussing what I should feed him.

7:06 pm: Quite looking forward to Bloke's arrival. Scheduling weirdness has meant that I've not actually seen him in a couple of weeks. Emails and phone aren't the same.

7:20 pm: He brought flowers! For our seventh anniversary. Which I confess, I had completely forgotten. My plan of a nice dinner was accidental, but quite convenient.

9:00 pm: Just finished a lovely dinner and couple of jokes with Bloke. We're playing video games.

11:00 pm: A shag that, for once, was not interrupted by my cats. Good times.

TUESDAY

6:45 am: Hear Bloke leaving to catch his train. Ah, my men all leave me so early.

11:00 am: Chatting to Hubby online. I've now been with him more than half my life. Not sure whether the relationship with Bloke will last quite that long – he may want to settle down with someone who can give him her full attention. At the moment it suits him to have a part-time relationship, but that may not last forever.

11:15 am: Hubby's talking about his girlfriend. She's religious, and I've never quite figured out how she squares an active sex life involving multiple partners with the teachings of her religion. But whatever floats her boat.

12:30 pm: A quiet morning, time to think of how things stand. One husband, one boyfriend. I'm happy with both, and have insufficient time with both.

6:28 pm: Just finishing up some work and chatting to Hubby online before he heads out for the evening. Me, I get to go to the ever-exciting gym. Be still, my heart.

9:45 pm: Back home from gym and irritable (knee hurting, bad class). I would like a little cuddle, but that's a non-starter: Bloke is 40 minutes away, and Hubby an hour flight. Considering a swift bitchfest email to Bloke.

11:00 pm: Dinner helps, somewhat.

11:35 pm: Decided against the email. Hubby is online and sympathetic about gym class.

—m—

the mum choosing between her husband and her ongoing one-night stand

29, FEMALE, SURREY

MONDAY

3:30 pm: Saw my Non-Boyfriend at work all day today where I handle accounts, and really wanted him. I'm currently sleeping with a work colleague, though no one knows.

4:15 pm: We had a quick snog in the elevator.

5:59 pm: At home. Just got an instant message from Non-Boyfriend at work, telling me what he would do to me if he were here with me. God, I'm really horny. Wish he was here. I feel guilty thinking about him.

6:05 pm: I am currently separated from my husband, though we still live and sleep together with our two young children. Non-Boyfriend knows I'm married/separated, but is falling deeper in love. We had a one-night stand seven months ago and never parted.

6:08 pm: Non-Boyfriend is on his way home and still telling me what he's going to do to me. I need a decision fast.

8:45 pm: Huge argument with the Non-Boyfriend. He's supposed to come over and see me, but he decided to do his ironing first. Saw him at work all day and really wanted him. Never sleep tonight.

8:53 pm: It's not even ten minutes, and I've already called him pretending I'm not angry. I just need a booty call, but he doesn't need to know that.

9:21 pm: Another row. No booty call. Since when does ironing prioritise over a fuck? So mad.

9:30 pm: Sigh. A couple of weeks ago, I popped round to his and got really drunk with him and his mate. He walked me home and I grabbed him at the gate and he fucked me hard against the fence. At first it was more lust, but then I started to fall for him. Oh shit, what am I going to do?

TUESDAY

6:58 am: Typical, I was asleep by the time the husband got home. I'm convinced the husband had cheated and is possibly fucking a work colleague, but would never admit it. He likes to be the bad boy and that's what I like. He knows we're separated but still sees me as his.

12:22 pm: Oh, what to do. The hubby is off today, should I make a quick stop home for lunch? Totally confused. I'm not sure if I'm married, single or in a relationship.

5:35 pm: Fell out with the Non-Boyfriend again over something stupid. He's being a pain in the arse and I'm too tired.

6:00 pm: Staying late at work. It's not really worth the hot sex, is it? Non-Boyfriend and I slept together by accident, after a work night out. He broke up with his girlfriend three weeks later. Our relationship works – it's just that all our time together is at work.

6:15 pm: He gets the good bits, he sees me dressed up for work, dressed for nights out. He gets the thrill of no one knowing, and he doesn't get the shit of shared bills, kids and arguing over the dishes.

8:00 pm: At Non-Boyfriend's house for a bit, laying on the bed, chatting for a while, just holding each other.

9:30 pm: We were supposed to head straight out, but we started kissing, and slowly it got hotter and hotter. I'd told him I didn't want to fuck, as I couldn't be bothered with the mess, but the odd thing is I really wanted him inside me. As I sat on top of him he grabbed my breasts, I could feel his hard cock pressing against me. We started kissing more intensely and I knew I had to go before I fucked him. So I just got up to go.

9:50 pm: That didn't work. Just went to leave, and he grabbed me from behind and pushed his hand down my trousers feeling for my knickers, pushing them to one side. He slid his fingers into my pussy, and I was already very wet. He started to slide his fingers inside and out, doing this thing he does that drives me wild. I came quickly.

9:55 pm: My phone is vibrating in my bag. It's my hubby wondering if I finished work and will be home to put the kids to bed. Oh fuck.

10:00 pm: Heading home, and feel quite ashamed as I let Non-Boyfriend get me off and left him with nothing.

WEDNESDAY

11:08 am: I'm working from home today. It's stressful, as I know my job's not permanent.

12:05 pm: Still not a word from the husband, he left at 6 am for work. Even though we're separated I would be gutted if he were with someone else, as would he. That's why I have to keep this a secret or end it. One or the other.

12:15 pm: Thinking about my hubby. He's the best relationship I've ever had. If I fight hard enough, I could be so happy. I've always felt as though he just went along with things: I was the one who suggested that we get engaged, that we move house, have kids.

1:30 pm: Non-Boyfriend is about to pop in on his lunch break. He's starting to annoy me with neediness. He seems to have to see me every day, and as his need is growing, my need is lessening.

2:00 pm: I told him that he has no fire in his belly, so he kissed me so hard that he bit and burst my lip. 'Fire,' I said, 'not crazy.'

2:19 pm: I can't imagine anything more boring than emailing the Non-Boyfriend all day.

5:33 pm: Another outing with my husband ruined. So mad. Husband called in a mood, saying I was out all the time and was never in.

5:38 pm: Emailed the Non-Boyfriend saying that I need some time on my own tonight. Getting stressed out.

7:20 pm: I think tonight's question should be, 'Who's let you down the most today?' Just had a general bad day, getting stressed out about work and the fact that my job isn't permanent. Just seem to get overlooked a lot at home/family. I seem to be the one who can't moan about problems as everyone else's seem more important.

11:11 pm: After no sympathy, I'm off to bed.

THURSDAY

9:32 am: Woke up late, and got to work to discover that not much had been done on my day off. Half two they finished, and spent the rest of the day on the Internet. Magic.

10:15 am: Arrrr. Hubby forgot to grab my lunch. Was good to see him mid-morning, even if he did forget my lunch. I really do love him, just not in the way I should.

3:30 pm: Huge fight with Non-Boyfriend at work. Over nothing as usual, just me feeling insecure about myself, mixed with the confusions of the relationship.

5:15 pm: Had a bad day at work and walked into the house looking a mess, sat and had a cry and picked myself up again.

7:14 pm: Spent the past two hours looking through the home computer history. I'm hurt that my hubby's been looking at porn again. I found a few items. A few years ago we had an incident when I found porn on my husband's phone, and he lied and said it was a mate showing him something. Then he made a mistake and subscribed to something on the computer, and I had to call them up and say it was only used by me and must've been an error. That finished me, I think. I realise I have trust issues.

8:10 pm: Challenged hubby on the items that I found. He denies it, and this used to be a shared computer. He says that the history was a bookmark rather than dates. I'm not averse to porn, to be honest it turns me on. But I'd rather watch it together. I feel so rubbish.

7:29 pm: Non-Boyfriend sent an email saying: *love you.* I felt ill when I saw it. I know I don't love him back and feel I'm stringing him along. I don't think I want either of them. I want to be me.

1:26 am: We broke up. I'm gutted, devastated. I didn't think I would be.

FRIDAY

8:45 am: New girl starts at work. She's sitting next to the Non-Boyfriend. Instant dislike. Bit gutted, as her job is the one I went for, but was told that I didn't have enough experience. Not happy. More instant dislike.

10:00 am: She has started to call me pet names when we're dealing with each other. More dislike.

10:05 am: Non-Boyfriend goes to make tea, I go with. He tells me how nice she is. We're still not really talking. He's trying to be nice but I'm in a mood. I hate her more.

1:35 pm: They have sat giggling all day. He knows I'm mad.

1:37 pm: At my desk, I can't be bothered today. Work colleague asks if I've been dumped. I give him a look, he says 'OMG, it would be *bad* if you had.' I give a laugh and pretend it's a joke. I could cry.

2:15 pm: Phone hubby at work. He makes a joke about needing time to himself. I hang up. Is he kidding? I cry at my desk, and blame hay fever – which I don't have.

4:30 pm: Non-Boyfriend and new girl call my name. I barely acknowledge him. Then I realise it's a line from a movie, *Up*, one that we joke about with the kids. It was our joke, now it's theirs – they can have it.

5:15 pm: The office starts to joke about how they are BFFs after just a day.

5:30 pm: Finally. I normally walk home in a group. Today I say I need to walk another route, give a bullshit reason. I walk home crying.

5:45 pm: At home, just asked hubby for a hug. He said he's busy. I cried, and told him I'm emotional and tired, and had a busy time at work. He buys it. Why not.

7:30 pm: In the bed with a bottle of wine. Locked the door, and plan to stay here singing sad songs till I'm very drunk.

10:20 pm: I'm drunk and tired in bed and almost asleep, so upset.

SATURDAY

5:30 am: I'm up and awake but hung-over. Work colleague off so I can't phone in sick. Plus most of Facebook knows I was drunk.

7:45 am: I'm in work. Stupid overtime. Stupid financial year-end.

8:15 am: I sit and ignore Non-Boyfriend when he says good morning.

8:30 am: In the kitchen, he says hello again. I ignore him further. Now back at my desk to a sarcastic email from him because I ignored him. I'm not in the mood.

11:16 am: I just emailed Non-Boyfriend to ask if he wants tea.

11:20 am: We went to the kitchen in silence, and I just came back to my desk and another email from him. He wants to know why I asked him to tea and said nothing.

11:22 am: I really wanted him to say something, but he didn't.

12:00 pm: Non-Boyfriend asks what I'm doing for lunch. I say nothing. No appetite – brilliant diet.

12:15 pm: He asks me to go for a walk with him.

12:30 pm: I agree.

12:45 pm: We're at the canal talking. I'm crying. At least we're talking again.

5:30 pm: Going home. Free. Thank God.

7:30 pm: Text message from the Non-Boyfriend. Do I want to go to a BBQ at his friend's house. Tomorrow?

SUNDAY

5:15 am: I'm awake, can't sleep. This dilemma is killing me. Do I dump my husband who I do love, just not in the way I should, or do I dump the Non-Boyfriend who I have a love/hate relationship with?

6:19 am: Jumped upon by kids. Time to be mum again. Will I get a chance to be me? I smile, I get breakfast and I break the news I am going out today.

2:35 pm: I'm in a car heading to London with the Non-Boyfriend and his two mates. They are very nice to me considering I'm the woman who stole him from his ex-girlfriend, who is their friend.

4:10 pm: I'm hideously drunk. I thought the best plan was to keep up with the boys. It worked. I can drink them under the table, but I didn't eat from the E. coli-ridden barbecue. I feel sick.

4:20 pm: I'm standing outside feeling sick. He just came up behind me. I think he only wants me for sex or arm candy.

10:30 pm: We have just fucked in the toilets. Classy. I initiated it. I pulled him in and started heavy kissing him and stripping before sucking his cock and grabbing him till he fucked me over the bath.

11:00 pm: I am in a car on my way home.

1:00 am: I'm home in bed, and stopped only to puke in the toilet. I got home to a, 'Hey baby, did you have fun? Sorry for being an arse earlier.' Bollocks. I feel shit.

—m—

5

REMARRIED, RECOMMITTED

the former salacious sixties man with a live-out wife and a viagra habit

75, MALE, LONDON

MONDAY

9:00 am: Every day, I try to take an hour's walk with the belief that it's good for me. Today accompanied by Officer Winston. He is a compulsive talker, and he escorts one like a faithful dog. He's a frightful bore, but he's such a curiosity that I find him quite engaging.

9:15 am: He regales me with his work. He spends every morning collecting the eclectic range of girls' cards down the high street, carefully filing them in a plastic-paged model book. Then he telephones the girls to say that what they're doing is illegal. 'You can't start before 2 pm or you wake them and they're pissed off.' In the early evening their pimps replace every card. He enjoys his job.

12:30 pm: Came home, had lunch and read the *Times*. My wife Miriam and I, we do meet quite frequently, but she has her own apartment in West London, and she meets me there more than not. I've been with her for 15 years and we've never lived together. Got married two years ago. Many relationships suffer from proximity, which rubs the edge off it. I see her at least once a week.

2:00 pm: Reading Jay McInerney's *The Good Life*. One of his characters remarks that a man has four needs: food, drink, pussy and strange pussy. How true. I'm surprised and grateful to find that, despite old age, I still have a keen interest in sex. And, thanks to those magical blue pills, if any woman is so gracious as to express an interest in my cock, I can still muster a creditable erection. Stamina is another matter. I do so miss coke and speed, the perfect accompaniment to advanced sex, but for the moment it's quite fun to stay alive.

6:00 pm: Came home, eating dinner. One of the reasons I don't go out to dinner parties is that a party which doesn't contain the potential of a sexual relationship is bloody dull. Until very recently I would flirt with any woman. But I've just read George Melly's book, and he said that one cannot flirt with younger women because it looks grotesque. He watched a tape of a show where he'd flirted with the 30-year-old presenter, and after that he resolved not to again. Very sound advice.

9:00 pm: Spoke to Miriam about my day. It's a week since we last met, though we speak often. She's as much a loner as myself and the arrangement works perfectly. The perils of cohabitation stifle even the best relationship and certainly affect desire.

9:30 pm: At least once or twice every ten days, we spend the night together. It works for us. One or the other of us will stay over at the other's flat. There's an absence of routine, routine is a killer in anything. Fortunately she nor I are the kind of people who want constant togetherness.

TUESDAY

10:00 am: This morning I captivated Winston with a story: when I was very much younger, I got a call in my office in Bond Street from my first wife (there have only been two), who said the flat was full of policemen. They came round in force expecting to find a dealer, and they found small quantities of everything. A recreational user in a steady job, I walked away with a £90 fine. I am more or less straight, depending on circumstance and the drugs being served.

10:05 am: The mid-1960s to late 1970s were the peak of my sexual adventures. Both my wife and myself were widely unfaithful to each other, but we understood. We did a lot of group sex in my first marriage. An orgy involves four people or more. Surely any lesser number is an intimate relationship. The women were wonderfully adventurous, but we, the men, were pretty uptight about showing interest in each other's erections. I regret we were so inhibited. Everyone would have had more fun if we'd been gayer.

10:07 am: These fond memories used to lead to masturbation. No longer; my sexual energies, such as they are, are well taken up by my marriage and the sex I'm fortunate enough to have.

11:14 am: Went to communion in central London, a thing that's stabilised my life and is at odds with the way I've lived much of it. I don't go to a local church because much of the Christian faith does a thing called neighbourliness, where you're asked to shake hands with everyone, and I can't stand it.

1:30 pm: Back from lunch with a television friend at The Garrick. Rather grand surroundings and nursery food. I tell him about Officer Winston and in return he tells me about a policeman they had on a night location years ago on *The Likely Lads*, who said that in his early days when homosexuality was illegal, he and another officer were assigned to 'cottage watch' above the notorious public lavatory in Regent's Park. They spent hours crouched in the crawl space below the roof, eyes glued to drilled holes below. The policeman said, 'You wouldn't believe the stuff you saw going on. When someone came in to take a shit it was like a breath of fresh air.'

3:00 pm: About to visit an old friend, Peter, in his new care home. His life ain't so bad, despite the fact he can no longer walk and three-quarters of his marbles are missing. Each morning he's hosed down and dressed. Put on his buggy, motors out to a pub lunch and two bottles of wine. He wears a sign saying where he lives.

4:15 pm: Today Peter showed me a new sex video. Even if not capable of physical expression, libido lives on in his head. He tells me of a club for special needs in King's Cross run by a handicapped pole-dancer and with wheelchair access. I refused to take him.

4:30 pm: Back home, I am now thinking how ungenerous of me. It's rather horrifying but the sexual impulse seems to last in the ghost in the mind, if not in the body, until an unsuitably and decrepit age. It's a fairly nasty idea. I do think sex should be restricted to under the age of 35, just because they look better.

4:35 pm: My sex life, thank God, is active enough. It is confined to my wife but, yes, I find it extremely satisfactory. I know a lot of people my age to have very unsatisfactory relationships and sex lives. I am lucky in choice, situation, health and capability.

8:00 pm: Home, reading about black propaganda in World War II. An honoured general has just died. The misinformation spread is that he had a heart attack while engaged in an orgy with his mistress and two sailors, wearing a spiked German helmet. One wouldn't really want to die like that. It would take some explaining to St Peter at the gate.

WEDNESDAY

9:00 am: Walking up the King's Road flanked by Winston and his partner, we're getting curious looks from passers-by. I realise people think that these two are personal protection officers. I have found the latest must-have accessory, madly sexy and status-enhancing. Wearing that pair, I couldn't fail to score.

1:00 pm: Damn good dinner with Miriam, talking about life and fresh subjects. As Cyril Connolly said, 'A particular charm of marriage is the dialogue, the permanent conversation between two people.'

1:03 pm: He also said, 'There is no more sombre enemy of good art than the pram in the hall.'

3:00 pm: I was walking down King's Road when a woman's voice says, 'Hello.' She was one half of a middle-aged couple sitting at a bus stop. I knew I'd met them, but couldn't place them. Buying time to recall them, I said, 'Oh how lovely to see you,' etc, etc. We talked for three or four minutes with animation and warmth, until their bus came. Moments later I realised it was my ex-wife and her husband. I hadn't seen her for ten years. Had I recognised her, I wouldn't have been nearly so nice.

5:54 pm: Stopped off to fill a prescription. I take Viagra whenever I'm promised a sexual encounter, about once a week. It does not stimulate the libido, but after a certain age, one's erection becomes much less forceful. It relaxes the veins so you can express yourself physically as you feel.

9:00 pm: Spoke to Miriam. She laughed when I told her about the bus stop. Miriam has been married to several of my friends – I'm her fourth husband. One can't live a while without being with someone who's been round the block. I hope she's my last wife. I would say she's the love of my life.

—⁓—

the welsh pensioner spending 24/7 with her second husband, tempted to unplug his tv

64, FEMALE, SOUTH WALES

MONDAY

10:59 am: Andrew brought me breakfast in bed and then massaged my feet. It's his way of showing he loves me. We've been married for 20 years. I know he loves me, but I wish he'd tell me occasionally or give me an actual hug.

11:27 am: Amy, the youngest of our eight combined children from previous marriages, just rang to tell me of relationship problems with her boyfriend. I wanted to say, 'Don't tell me, I don't have all the answers.' Andrew hardly looks at me or touches me spontaneously. He's comfortable and content, while I wish for more. I didn't say that.

2:00 pm: Andrew's friend Wynton arrived. He flirted with me and made me laugh, Andrew doesn't seem to notice, he's too busy watching TV. They're in their seventies and I'm 64, so it's all innocent. Andrew and I are like Tweedledum and Tweedledee, rotund (he has a large belly, I have a large bosom), and we squabble a lot about silly things.

3:30 pm: My single, 40-year-old daughter came to visit. We talked about her bad choices in men. I have a husband who loves me, and that should be enough.

10:20 pm: Bed. Andrew's downstairs watching TV. It will be hours before he joins me. But when I wake in the night as I often do, there'll be a cup of chocolate on the bedside table for me.

TUESDAY

12:00 pm: On the bus to town for weekly bill paying. Both of us are always tense when we go out. He is an extrovert, drawing attention to himself, and I'm embarrassed. It's my problem, not his. He doesn't like waiting in queues, gets really snappy and impatient. I hire a mobility scooter and try to do as many things as possible while he waits in the bank. Staying with him can be a nightmare.

2:15 pm: Arrived home with a takeaway meal. On the bus we joked with each other, him pressing his leg against mine, and mine pressing back, like isometric exercise. Was my leg really stronger than his, or was he just letting me win?

6:15 pm: Just made love. Not hours of acrobatics like we used to. Now that we're older and less fit, half an hour is pushing it. Andrew doesn't take Viagra, but we've agreed if it's necessary he will. But really, I just like the cuddling up and physical closeness. He always says, 'I could do this every day,' but in reality, he doesn't. We have sex three or four times a month, sometimes five. All in all, I'm lucky.

6:20 pm: In my first marriage, which lasted a quarter-century, I never had an orgasm, and my husband would keep asking – Are you? Have you? Did you? I felt so pressured. I don't want Andrew to feel like that. I just want to be with him. Sex with Andrew is more exciting, animal-like and rougher. It's more 'raw sex' than 'loving.'

6:25 pm: In his defence, my first husband tried everything possible to make me have an orgasm – positions, toys, dressing up – so I've done almost everything you can think of: sadism, masochism, bondage, golden rain, etc. I do still wonder what a lesbian relationship would be like.

8:00 pm: A call from one of my daughters to tell me that one of her druggie friends died. I find it hard to be sympathetic, which isn't very nice. She has been a registered addict for many years, she takes methadone.

11:00 pm: Andrew's watching TV, and we've had a lovely day. I love Andrew. Perhaps he can only express love by doing things for me. Off to bed.

WEDNESDAY

11:08 am: Off to my writing group with my friend Angela. My arthritis (in my spine, pelvis, neck, knees and hips – I have a walking stick and can't stand long) is mild compared to hers. I don't think she and her husband have sex any more. We make lots of jokes and innuendos about sex, but there's a line we don't cross: the truth.

12:30 pm: Good writers' meeting. One woman, Mary, is 83 and a spinster. In her 20s she fell in love with a man whose wealthy parents gave him a choice: Mary or your inheritance. He chose the latter, and Mary has been writing about unrequited love ever since.

4:29 pm: Jonny, a 14-year-old music pupil of mine, just left. He has acne popping out, his voice is squeaky. I don't have any toyboyish fantasies, but I can see that he has those 'come to bed' eyes, and will have the girls after him when he's older.

4:31 pm: I think I must be really immature because the best relationship I ever had was with a boy when I was 15. We didn't have sex. More often than not we wrestled together, and would always kiss goodnight. We used to just talk and laugh. I just want someone to flirt with me and make me laugh. Not 'someone'. Andrew.

5:00 pm: Andrew's brother Jeffrey and I are eating cake. Jeffrey divorced 20 years ago, and was quite a womaniser. He always listens as if I'm the only one in the room, and buys me something feminine (perfume) for Christmas. (Andrew gives me money and tells me to get something I want.) I used to fancy him, but don't at all now, though my youngest daughter thinks he fancies, if not loves, me.

5:07 pm: This is relevant because I had an affair with my first husband's brother. My ex-husband encouraged it, saying he felt sorry for his brother, and that God wants us to share our love – but what he really wanted was to be a voyeur. It didn't turn out the way he wanted. Once or twice a week for two years, his brother would come over and my ex would go to church (really!). I fell in love with the brother (and yes, I did orgasm), and our marriage ended. Now my ex and I are polite, as if we've never known each other. I talk more to his wife. And the brother's wife, whom I have known for 50 years and see regularly, is totally unaware. I live in fear that one day she will find out. There are no excuses.

6:01 pm: Upstairs with loads of emails, letters and photocopying to do – I'm a retired cashier, this should be easy! We seem to fluctuate between being two people who live in the same house, as now when I'm upstairs and he's down, and being two people that people assume as one, so much so that people automatically ask after the other. I think we've adapted to being 24/7 the best we can.

8:30 pm: I think he really is a TV addict. I'm bored. The wall he has built around himself is very strong.

11:10 pm: Doing the online grocery shopping. Years ago Andrew would sneak up and kiss my neck and one thing would lead to another. Now TV is more interesting to him, and I've lost the will to go seduce him. At our age, spirit is willing, flesh is weak. It took a good few years for me to get the message: TV first, sex after. I feel sad thinking of all the wasted hours, the fact that we're getting older and don't know what's in front of us. But hand on my heart, it's not intercourse I long for: it's a non-sexual cuddle, a non-asked-for kiss, an 'I love you' without me saying it to him first.

THURSDAY

9:30 am: Woke up a lot through the night. Andrew is his usual happy self, not realising what's going on. Why am I complaining? It is an 'alive' day.

11:05 am: Showered, feel better. Andrew went to the post office, just shouted, 'See you!', no kiss goodbye.

11:45 am: House to myself, masturbated. I have typical latent guilty feelings, the results of strict upbringing and ignorance, and disloyalty to Andrew. Only when totally by myself can I be me in every way. Feel unsettled.

1:15 pm: Just rowed with Andrew. He brought fish and chips back for lunch, which I thought was kind until I asked for the change from the post office, and he said he'd bought second-class stamps rather than first, so that there was money for the meal.

1:25 pm: He's sulking and I'm fuming! I now have to phone people and explain why they won't get the post tomorrow. Seems petty, and it probably is, but in my ever-decreasng world, it's enormous!

3:14 pm: Have calmed down now. Andrew's just brought me tea, and he is hoovering. He never says 'sorry,' so we never make up – it just passes. I make up all kinds of reasons for him not saying sorry rather than actually discuss it with him.

3:18 pm: I suppose the hovering and cup of tea *is* his way of making up. I'll go downstairs and kiss his bald head and cuddle later on.

3:20 pm: Even rowing seems exciting sometimes. Is it weird of me to think that? When we row, I am seeing the real him.

4:15 pm: Oh no! Now we're back to where we were. He asked me to make single photocopies, which I just did, and now he's saying he asked for two. 'No, you didn't!' 'Yes, I fucking did… ' He's grumpy, I'm fuming.

7:28 pm: Normality's resumed. He's downstairs watching TV and I'm upstairs. I'll go downstairs in a minute and join him for an evening of TV, and at least we'll be together, which is more than some people have.

10:30 pm: I normally wait until the adverts are on to speak, but he was channel-hopping, so I spoke. He irritatedly said, 'What?' I said, 'Oh please don't make me say it again,' and he exploded into a tirade that ended with, 'And don't you ever make *any* mistakes?!' (Yes, but I admit them.) So now we're not talking, and I'm going to bed. Totally childish, but I've tried everything else. If he dies before me I'm burying the TV with him!

FRIDAY

6:30 am: Andrew is heavier and bigger than me and kept turning over, almost pushing me out of bed several times. We're both deaf without our hearing aids, and I have arthritis, so the most I could do was try to push him unsuccessfully away.

10:38 am: Woke up with a migraine, and Andrew massaged my feet, especially the big toe, which is supposed to help. Went back to sleep.

1:40 pm: Yesterday was definitely not a good day. I know he loves me, but it's not enough. Is it because he doesn't show it? Or am I a self-pitying cow?

4:15 pm: Worried that one of my daughters is in a controlling relationship. I used to be like that, because of being in a controlling situation for a long time – you go into defensive victim mode. I hope she doesn't play the submissive part, even when she doesn't have to.

7:20 pm: Just finished watching a DVD with Andrew, it was a good film and we both enjoyed it, which is quite rare as we have very different tastes. We shared it, and it felt good. Which at our age is the best we could hope for. He has never been what I imagine a soulmate to be, but he is the other half of my heart, and I want to spend every minute of my life as part of his.

—⚬—

WHEN RELATIONSHIP BECOMES LIFESTYLE

6

PARENTS OF CHILDREN

the happily horny, heavily pregnant journalist

27, FEMALE, LONDON

THURSDAY

7:59 am: Used a hypnosis CD to get to sleep last night. Worked a treat. Being a half-whale makes sleep more difficult, and I struggle to switch my mind off. We're expecting our first child in four weeks, and I flit between excitement and sheer terror.

8:15 am: Nice cuddle this morning. We are both working in the City today, separately, and he always gets nervous something will happen to me.

8:37 am: Self-love. Not that I was feeling horny – Radio 4 was on for Christ's sake. I just needed to prove to myself that I am still capable of such things. That I'm more than a human incubator. Feel a tinge of sadness that in a few weeks' time, that part of my anatomy will be unrecognisable. It's a bit like saying goodbye to a treasured old friend.

10:15 am: Train. Finding myself ogling the ample thigh of the young, chubby woman opposite. The rhythm of the train shifts her short hemline around her waist. I am fixated on this thigh, with an urge to bite it, sink my fingers into the doughy flesh. It's not a sexual urge, just attraction to the proud fleshiness, the arrogance of being fat and sensual. I don't possess that gorgeous sexuality.

10:17 am: Baby kicks me to say, 'Stop perving, you're a mother now.'

3:59 pm: Feeling my identity as a hard-working, erudite professional slip away. Colleagues have started to use a different voice to address me, all soft and gooey, like there is an invisible baby already in my arms.

10:33 pm: No energy to talk politics with Other Half, with whom I am still madly in love after five years.

11:00 pm: Upstairs for shower and the dreaded 'perineal massage'. This is misleading: it is neither a massage nor particularly limited to that area of your anatomy, if the textbook is to be believed. The book advises that six weeks before birth you begin to prepare your perineal area by stretching it until it stings and holding it there for a minute. I bought the special oil online because I was too embarrassed to buy it in the shop. But will do anything to avoid needing stitches.

11:10 pm: The diagram is not entirely clear and I am still confused how this is meant to work. Blergh.

FRIDAY

9:48 am: A rare lie-in together. Talked about how our relationship will change. I feel I've played my evolutionary trump card now, so all the sex and love of the last few years will probably go. 'No,' he says, 'now I get to watch you become a wonderful mother.' Which sounds great for friends, but for a lover?

10:02 am: Says Other Half: 'I was thinking last night how we've been together all these years and I still love you to bits.' I well up. Two months ago I was an emotional yo-yo. I panicked that I wasn't bonding with the baby, and warned Other Half that I would leave him with the baby at the hospital and run away. But now I am programmed to be calm and positive. Oxytocin is pumping around my body to prepare for labour and bond me to the sperm-provider.

11:01 am: I'm not religious, but been thinking about the Virgin Mary. Her virginity seems a convenient solution to the conflict as you move from girlfriend/lover/wife to mother. Maybe the virgin tale has been perpetuated for centuries because it's a good way that mothers can still be sexual beings; the husband is still happy that nothing is being taken away from him. Motherhood doesn't mean you have to be pure and good from now on.

12:25 pm: Birth pool we ordered for home water birth arrives. It comes with a sieve. No human process should ever require a sieve. No wonder I'm concerned about the romance going.

4:09 pm: He's out of sorts. I suggest some *things* we could do to improve his mood, but he is very huggy and clingy as he leaves for work. 'I'm sorry, I don't know what it is,' he says. 'I love you.' He kisses my belly 'And I love you, Baby.' Already? Do I?

4:11 pm: What if I love the baby more than him? What if I don't love the baby and go mental and he sees me differently? What if we stop loving each other?

6:58 pm: Other Half home with ice cream for me. He didn't have one for himself. He only had a pound left after grocery shopping and he used it to get me an ice cream. That's romance.

9:07 pm: Sorted out the house. We make such a good team. With the exception of a few days here and there, we have basically spent 24 hours a day together for five years working mostly from home. We are good like that.

SATURDAY

10:02 am: Sad dream in which, on a never-ending foreign coach journey, I watch Other Half fall in love with an erudite Penelope Cruz.

1:34 pm: Went back to bed mid-morning and spent the hours napping, making love, napping, making love. *Amazing.* 'Thought you weren't doing "naughty" any more,' he grins. Seems mothers are capable of Cartesian separation after all. Relief!

1:45 pm: He gets out of bed and says, 'All of that can't be good for the baby.' I tell him not to think about the baby. 'It's pretty hard not to.'

5:57 pm: Put up bunting in nursery. He looks a bit freaked out; it's becoming a proper reality now.

6:57 pm: Just watched Rachel's unrealistic birth on *Friends*. Led to an impromptu test on what should have happened, which we both passed with flying colours. He's so clued up, he could be a midwife.

6:59 pm: Heading out now to a lecture about covert operations in everyday society. Yes, I know we are dull.

10:54 pm: Back from a dreamy date: excellent, interesting lecture followed by dinner at our favourite restaurant with stimulating conversation and a reminder we are both adults. Feel very loved-up.

SUNDAY

10:31 am: He says, 'You're big but you're beautiful!' I only just realised that I am hugely, bovinely pregnant.

2:26 pm: Rearranging the kitchen. The world is full of meaningless stuff, and we are about to be sucked into owning some of it. Accept that we are 27 going on 40.

4:22 pm: In the car, talking about how much we enjoyed our 'date' last night. He warns me that if we were ever to split up, not many men would find a lecture on national security sexy.

7:20 pm: My hospital bag has been packed for three months – and I'm not even going to hospital. When I think about the birth, I unpack everything and re-pack. Sort of helps. I have a tiny cry and admit that I feel quite scared. He reassures me, but I know he is also on edge.

9:37 pm: Fell asleep on his lap on the couch. A documentary was on about polygamous families. It kind of riles the feminist in me. I know I couldn't be happy.

MONDAY

10:18 am: I am looking forward to returning to cuddling up when we go to sleep. The whole time I've been pregnant, we've basically slept at far ends of the bed. Partly because I require a mountain of cushions, but mainly because he is so scared that he will accidentally bump or jolt my belly in the night. It must be like sleeping with a giant egg.

2:00 pm: My delight in coming home to find a new hoover gives way to depression. Twenty-seven and excited about the prospect of a special pet-hair nozzle. Not that long ago, I was partying for days on end in London warehouses, running around Soho with hookers, kissing girls, kissing boys, sleeping with friends. A lot of my friends came from London's underbelly – prostitutes, addicts, illegal immigrants. We would meet at three or four in the morning after work and get cabs to strange parties in weird places. The London bombing changed a lot of it. Someone close to me was involved, and it made me realise I wasn't living the life I wanted. I love having a stable life, albeit dull, but sometimes I get nostalgic for dysfunction.

5:55 pm: Back from another interesting lecture about the state of literature. Knackered. Going to play the pregnancy card and laze on the couch with the cats and a cream cake.

6:45 pm: Looking up 'lotus births'. For those unfamiliar, it involves keeping the baby, placenta and umbilical cord intact after birth until the cord naturally drops off. Other Half nearly vomits at the photo of a mum bathing a lotus baby.

9:00 pm: We watched half a Hitchcock movie, with a strange dynamic between an uncle and young niece, which to our 21st-century eyes seemed rather sinister and unsettling. I guess this is a sign of our sexualising times. The most unconvincing word today is 'platonic'. No one believes that word, I don't think.

TUESDAY

8:15 am: Get to work early to make my desk nice for the girl who'll be replacing me.

10:00 am: Training going well. She's bright and I like her. Her face isn't very pretty but she has a great figure and I kind of envy her svelte body and intact 'downstairs'. I divide women into two categories: those who have been bovine and scarred by childbirth, and those who haven't.

10:39 am: Make list of people to email when the child arrives. Quite a few exes on there. What will they feel when they get the email? Do they see me as 'The One That Got Away'? Or will they think, 'Phew, that was a lucky escape!' Hope Other Half tells his exes. Show them I've won. The whole time I've been pregnant I've been hoping to bump into his ex, but it has sadly not transpired. I'm sure it'll happen one day, so I hope the child is an angelic-looking heart-melter.

2:34 pm: Local café is chock full of prams and screaming, mewling newborns. Euch, what a horrendous din. Just get me one of the cute quiet ones off the adverts. The mums all looked pretty normal, though, not bovine or blobby.

5:00 pm: Am now officially on maternity leave. Let the thumb-twirling begin.

5:30 pm: Antenatal class, the time of the week when I hear every word I can't say myself repeated over and over for 90 minutes. I am plunged into the profoundly uncomfortable world of unmentionables. There's nowhere to hide – the walls are crammed with graphic, life-size photos of naked women in various stages of labour. Shudder.

8:13 pm: Back. Highlights included how to eat your placenta, and a live performance of what a contraction looks like.

8:15 pm: I am going to set up an antenatal class for repressed women. No disappointed looks when you admit that you haven't done any yoga and are baffled by perineal massage. No talk of the V-word.

8:51 pm: Other Half teases me about marriage. Sounds like he is less averse to the idea, maybe because I have laid off the idea. Maybe it's the pull of a Tory incentive.

11:20 pm: Other Half stepped out to see a gig, came home pleased to see me. Heading upstairs now. You'd have thought that at over eight months pregnant, there'd be some sort of health and safety procedure for lovemaking, but it remains surprisingly spontaneous, though sex now resembles not overcoming a quivering doe, but harpooning a beached whale. So on that note, good night folks.

the single dad away at sea, in love with a married woman

26, MALE, THE NORTH SEA

SATURDAY

5:00 am: Alarm has just woken me from a light slumber. I guess the time to go away has come again – back to my job as a merchant navy officer. I don't really want to go; the tearful goodbyes last night didn't help. I'm wondering if Jade, the girl I've become wrongly besotted by, will keep in touch while I'm gone? I really hope so.

7:52 am: Airport. I'm anxious. I miss home and my daughter. I refuse to cry in the departure lounge. There'll be time for that later, in private.

8:25 am: Sat waiting to board. Thinking about texting with Jade last night. She really cheered me up. Don't think she realises how a simple message from her makes me smile so wide.

9:09 am: Cruising high above the English coast, just over South Shields. I nodded off after take-off. She's in my dreams as well. I feel so stupid for getting this attached.

12:50 pm: Safely on-board the ship, and happier now that I've had a text from Jade. Her calling me 'bby' always makes me smile. I know it's wrong to hold any hope of a meaningful relationship with her, as I knew she was too good to be true: she has a partner.

7:15 pm: Done with work for the day, back on at 3 am. I'm absolutely shattered, I haven't eaten since breakfast. No appetite. Jade is texting me about an argument she's had with her husband. I know it's wrong, but their arguments only serve to give me hope.

8:01 pm: Texting quite graphically with Jade about masturbation. It began with me talking about how thin the walls are in my new cabin, and suddenly she is talking about needing to be quiet while she masturbates.

8:09 pm: Now she's telling me how she likes to be noisy and prefers toys. I'm really turned on now.

9:30 pm: We're texting about the stars and navigation; and now about how special she is.

SUNDAY

2:43 am: Awake and ready for my first early-morning watch. We work six hours on, six hours off – though shifts can sometimes stretch to eight or nine hours. Didn't get much sleep, as I chose to continue texting Jade before we sailed and lost the signal. Her partner is home today after working away. This makes me anxious that she won't message as much.

6:26 am: Morning watch completed. It was three hours of looking at the stars and thinking of last night's conversation with Jade. Excited for the day ahead, hoping she'll message me, and hoping I'll get to speak to my daughter on satellite phone. Her mum is pregnant. This doesn't trouble me; what does is that my daughter calls the husband's mum 'Grandma'. That hurts. It feels like she'll be calling him 'Dad' next. I couldn't handle that.

6:39 am: Aroused by some thoughts of Jade masturbating flashing through my mind. Wondering if it's wrong to masturbate to some videos she sent me when things were going ahead? After all the pictures, videos and sexual text messages, I would have liked to have actually put them all into practice.

11:40 am: Busy morning's work. There's a message waiting on Facebook from Jade. That pleases me no end. I've got a few hours before the next job starts so I'm going to sleep and deal with those arousing thoughts from earlier. They've been distracting me all morning.

1:35 pm: Just woke up from a power nap, after dealing with my urges. Couldn't help thinking about Jade while masturbating. Deep down inside I know it's wrong, but she really is all over my mind. Really not sure what to do. Maybe I should just stop talking to her. No I couldn't do that, I really value her as a friend despite my lust for more.

1:38 pm: Jade is showing as 'online' on Facebook, so I've just said hello. No reply, which saddens me. It all started this way, on a quiet Saturday night. She's an old schoolmate, and I'd been enjoying her status updates for weeks, and decided to say hello on chat. We got talking, and I felt that I could open up immediately. Now, it sounds trivial, but I really don't usually tell anybody about myself. So after a decade of not speaking, we had a really good long chat about our hopes, our lives, our children. It sounds ridiculous but I fell for her immediately.

1:40 pm: Our conversation that night soon became sexual. We'd both had a few glasses of wine. My phone burst into life, and I was over the moon to find a very sexual video. Things like this just don't happen to me. So that was the beginning of Jade and me. Things progressed quickly for a few weeks, but she has a partner and after a few weeks she decided she couldn't deal with the guilt. I'd let myself get attached, and now she is constantly on my mind.

5:05 pm: Just came down off the bridge after the afternoon's job. Back up in 20 minutes. Really missing home now. I would give anything to be there with my daughter, my family and my friends. I'm sat messaging them. Nothing from Jade. Really not a happy bunny right now.

6:31 pm: All smiles again. Message from Jade. Thank God my day is done! It all starts again at midnight.

7:04 pm: While in the shower, was pondering that Jade is home right now with her husband. Later on they will probably be having sex. This doesn't bother me in itself. You'd think I'd be jealous, but I'm not. Not of him, anyway. Just distressed that it will never be me.

MONDAY

1:17 am: Just had my call to tell me that the next job will be starting in 30 minutes. I was dreaming about Jade. In my dream we were talking, face-to-face. I can't remember much, but what sticks out was her saying, 'I have so much to tell you.'

6:43 am: Down from the bridge after a boring morning. It's one of the downsides to this job: periods of absolute chaos followed by long spells of boredom. I sat trying to convince myself that I should just give up hope of Jade. Now sat chilling for 20 minutes before I'm up again. No messages from anybody.

6:53 am: Just thought this: it's been *two* years since my last meaningful relationship ended. It was good while it lasted, about six months with a friend, parting mutual. But I don't like that thought at all. Two years seems like a lot of time to lose.

11:10 am: Mid-morning nap, strange dreams. No messages. A simple hello means so much out here.

11:25 am: I've just spoken to my mum and dad. My mum can be – how to put it? – *very vocal* about her opinions of my girlfriends. This can be a good thing and also a very bad thing. I admit that at times I have thought to myself 'What would mum say about Jade?' All seems well there, now off to lunch.

6:22 pm: Feeling much better after a good night's sleep. Working at sea has given me so much over the years (it's how I met my daughter's mum), but slowly killed my relationships. Up until the whole thing with Jade started, I was quite happy to plod along through life waiting for love to show itself. She has knocked me off my stride.

6:50 pm: All showered and smiling. I know, emotional roller coaster.

7:21 pm: Once again it's time for a film and sleep. Hopefully tomorrow I'll feel as calm as I do right now. What would happen if I just ignored Jade for a week or so? It goes against everything I stand for. Would she even notice? Could I manage it? There is only one way to find out.

TUESDAY

2:08 am: Alarm. Awoke every hour, but feel okay for the moment. My dreaming has reduced over the past few days, as has my sex drive and urge to self-pleasure. This is normal when I'm on-board. I'm not sure if everybody else is the same, but on-board, sex is something that drops off the radar. The other day was quite unusual and brought on by Jade.

2:15 am: The ship is rolling quite heavily. My Facebook inbox is alive, with messages from friends, family and… Jade. I actually thought, 'I hope there isn't anything from Jade.' Maybe I'm dying for her to cut me off. Painful, but for the best. Her note is short and sweet: *Hope you are okay? I'm a lil drunk, will write tomorrow. xoxo.* It's nice to know I crossed her mind.

2:20 am: Another message from my closest female friend, Harriet. We've spent a lot of time talking about Jade, who she knows. She discouraged me from getting involved. She's telling me to try and forget her, while noting how hard it is. She has always been right on this topic.

3:14 am: On bridge watch. Seven metre waves and 45 knot winds. Every time I look out to do some navigation by the stars, I think of Jade. I'm now regretting texting about the stars with Jade, opening myself up for more torture. The sad thing is that I really love opening up to Jade.

5:09 am: Dawn is breaking. Sat in my bridge chair thinking about commonalities in my relationships. My daughter's mum and I started similarly: She was dating another bloke who was treating her badly, so I took it upon myself to 'save' her. Similarities to Jade: She already has a husband? Check. It's complicated? Check. He treats her badly? Check. I really shouldn't be chasing after her? Check.

6:34 am: Something very strange has just come over me. All of a sudden my mind jumped to the first time I kissed Jade. It was amazing at the time, now it just leaves me gut-wrenched that I will never taste those sweet lips again. She instigated it, but I was very open to it, though I knew it could lead to no good.

8:05 am: Watching an American TV show about vampires. Made me think that maybe I'm approaching the whole Jade thing from the wrong angle. Maybe I should just back off and see what happens. That way I won't lose a friend, and maybe absence will make her heart grow fonder. I shouldn't take advice from the TV.

8:08 am: I'm doing a rubbish job of not thinking about her.

8:34 am: Back from breakfast a little late, and there's an email from my dad to say that my daughter's mum has given birth. As much as I wish her well, this news means nothing to me. Our relationship lasted a good number of years, loving, supportive and sexual, until she betrayed me. But it gave me my precious daughter, and she is the figurehead around which I rotate my life.

11:44 am: Power nap. The ship is rolling like mad, which makes everything more tiring. Moving around is difficult. Forcing myself to eat the peas rolling around my plate, as no real appetite. Still no message from Jade after she told me she would.

3:45 pm: Argh! Sat in my cabin thinking. I hate the fact that my life pretty much goes on hold while I'm away. I can't build any meaningful relationships, I lose out on time with my daughter, and I miss even silly things like wanting to sort new carpets.

3:48 pm: It's just occurred to me that when my relationship with my daughter's mum started, I had a fair range of female friends who could have become more. Compared to now it's quite sad really. All have since moved on, most into happy long-term relationships.

4:00 pm: Phone has sprung to life with a message from Jade. Excited even though I don't want to be.

4:10 pm: Message not worth getting excited for. Very short. Felt the need to keep my reply short, straightforward and without any emotion. I'm starting to see that her messages lengths depend on whether her husband is there. All I want is honest love. No bells and whistles. Just an honest girl with whom I spend forever with.

6:27 pm: I'm a little concerned about a dull ache in one of my testicles. Just checked myself over. It's a little alarming, and looking it up on Google was scary! Will decide later if it needs to be checked.

7:11 pm: Laid in bed watching the waves crash over my porthole, until an old school friend on Facebook chatted with me. She's being quite flirty, and so am I. I saw her on a night out last week. We had a chat and a dance and a good night kiss. I seem to have a thing for rekindling old school friendships at the moment.

8:31 pm: Just spent an hour talking, and really enjoyed it. We got cut short because my Internet went off, but I got a nice message saying was going to go put her kids to bed and then she'd be back to chat more. I want so much to have someone to come home to at the end of my sea trips.

—m—

the housewife trapped by a bipolar partner and two kids

43, FEMALE, DEVON

SATURDAY

9:13 am: My partner has taken our ten-year-old daughter to London. I keep getting excited texts. I'm thrilled for her. At the same time, I'm jealous that in 16 years together, he never took me to London. I realise this is because I was undemanding. My daughter fought for this, and she deserves it.

9:15 am: The last time our daughter was due to go to London, she packed her bag the night before and emptied her piggy bank to take her savings with her. Then my partner had the worst bout of illness he'd had (the doctors took him off antidepressants cold turkey – fun!), and he was so ill he didn't want to live. I was up all night with him. The moment when she unpacked her bag and put her money back was possibly the saddest moment of my life. My partner was very upset too; he'd let her down.

9:23 am: So I'm alone here with my six-year-old son till Sunday. He's good company, if a bit demanding. He refuses to let me go anywhere without following me. He can't stand being on his own, and I can't stand always being around other people. Not a good combination.

9:58 am: The flowers I bought for myself have died.

10:01 am: Gotta stop feeling sorry for myself. It's not that I'm lonely. Just not coping. I'm stuck at home with two kids and a long-term partner with bipolar disorder. Did I mention he's a closet transvestite? Normal would be lovely.

1:18 pm: How can I find him attractive, after everything he's done to make our lives so difficult? All that money gone. All the mood swings making our life so miserable.

1:20 pm: What am I talking about? I have a show I wrote being staged next week, just one of the few chosen to be performed. I should be proud of myself.

1:48 pm: I wish I could just go back to bed with a vibrator for half-an-hour. Cheer myself up. My son is bouncing on the sofa and wants me to keep him company.

3:00 pm: I wish I could talk to Peter about all of this. Talking to him, even on the phone, makes me feel alive again. Imagining myself away from here, where my identity returns, brings my libido back. Peter. We met at college, had a mad affair, then spent two years not managing to get together. A great loss in my life.

6:05 pm: Listening to all the wonderful things other park parents did with their kids this Easter holidays. I looked after a violently ill, suicidal man for three weeks.

9:45 pm: I wish Peter were not so far away. Even if I could just get on the phone to him. But he has to remain a secret. My kids would forever blame me for the split. Peter is my past, and I can't let that interfere with my present.

10:00 pm: My son sleeps with me. My partner and I sleep in separate rooms, have done for years. But in the mornings, when I'm horny, I really wish he was Peter.

SUNDAY

8:50 am: My six year-old is kicking a football at my legs.

8:55 am: I'm so glad I didn't marry my partner. He once asked me in a letter, ten years in. Apparently the look of horror on my face was enough for him to know that I would never marry him. Years ago I knew I wasn't happy, but then his poor mother was dying – she took so long to die! And then our first child came along (an accident!), and there just didn't seem to be the right time to leave.

9:01 am: I have mixed feelings about collecting my partner and our daughter tonight. I'd love to be the one getting on the train. I wished I lived a bohemian lifestyle, doing my paintings in a loft studio somewhere, with my bed unmade in the corner. When I paint my partner complains I'm making a mess.

4:47 pm: My partner just disappeared to his room to 'recover' from his trip. How much do you need to recover from a ten-year-old girl?

6:21 pm: My partner's occupational health report arrived. It confirms that he is now registered as disabled. Hit him like a brick, his mood plummeted. He is so tired now and so often in pain – his back, his neck, his stomach. We all end up walking on eggshells to prevent him from getting upset. It's like the problem is ours, not his. It's hard to say this, but we'd all be better off if he was dead.

8:09 pm: My partner is in such a bad state that he asked if we could have a 'session.' Sex. Not in a fun, just-wearing-normal-women's-clothes kind of way. He's into a bit of S&M, which after so many years is just so boring and unromantic.

10:15 pm: So a session entails: after the kids are asleep, he goes to his room and he dresses up in a big pink baby-doll outfit complete with a bonnet and pink gloves, and after ten minutes I come up and tie both his hands behind his back. I'm supposed to tease him a little, as though I'm the mistress forcing him to dress up like that, like he's my feminised slave. I'm getting bored just typing this. I just left him there struggling on the bed for 20 minutes or so. I suppose I should get all dressed up like an S&M mistress in black basque and stockings or something, but I'm just downstairs, making myself a cup of tea. Twenty minutes of peace in the evening is nice.

10:45 pm: So I went back up, teased him some more, undid some of his clothes and gave him a hand job. He's on antidepressants, which make it difficult for him to orgasm any other way, so I do it as a service.

10:52 pm: We last had intercourse when my son was conceived. And it wasn't that good! I dread the sessions now. I always do them if he asks – hell, it's no trouble really. But sometimes he asks three or four times a week now, and that invades my time a bit.

MONDAY

7:50 am: Getting my partner to work. I get him tea and cereal, find his hairbrush, get his clothes, check a bandage. I've got a decaying old man living in my house. I feel nothing for him. I think I'm going to have to yell at his doctor. We can't go on like this.

8:30 am: He left. I don't think he's fit to be at work. Certainly not fit to drive. He collapsed at work four years ago, then again last year – just had a breakdown in front of the hundreds of staff he administrates. If he collapses again, he's likely to lose his job, and I'll end up unable to work because I'm looking after him. But then what work could I do anyway? I left a good job, and I've been looking after the kids for nearly ten years now.

9:15 am: I have the next six hours to myself. Yippee! After doing my duty yesterday, I feel I deserve some time to write.

1:10 pm: The post! My excitement for the day. There is a letter for my partner offering him an 'emergency' appointment with the psychotherapist… for next month. After discovering he'd spent over £10,000 on credit cards I now open all the mail.

1:37 pm: Thinking about Peter. When I was 23, I seduced him and we had great, horny, dirty sex. I couldn't walk properly the following day. Just the sight of him made me horny, the touch of his skin, the hard muscles beneath – I just lost it. I had to have him. But he was engaged to someone else. He was very sorry – a drunken lapse – and I was very nice about it. But I shouldn't have been nice about it. I should have stolen him away. I look back and realise that was a defining moment of my life now.

1:39 pm: At one time we were in touch every day, sometimes at night when everyone else was asleep. After the birth of my son, for years I enjoyed the secret emails and texts, writing little scenarios to turn him on. He's stuck too, the dutiful father. They don't have sex anymore either. So here we are, good, responsible people, when all we want is a dirty weekend together. When was the last talk? Months ago, on the phone. And we laughed so much.

8:29 pm: Back from the park. Lots to do tonight. My partner said very little, ate, went to bed. My daughter got herself to bed. She shouldn't have to. At ten years old, bedtime is still a special time.

9:51 pm: So do you want to hear more about Peter? I sure do. Just typing his name makes me excited. We met again at a college reunion, him with a hard body beneath his T-shirt. I wanted him right there. Just the sound of his voice made me horny. But I was already four months pregnant with my second child. The look of disappointment on his face when I told him.

TUESDAY

8:30 am: In partner's room. Transvestite men have absolutely terrible taste in women's clothes. He used to love buying me clothes. I thought he was being affectionate. Now I realise it was the clothes he secretly wanted to wear. Once he took me to a dress store, and kept bringing out these big pink outfits for me to try.

10:26 am: My partner made it to work, but he's very ill. So here's the plan. A bit of success, a bit of losing weight. I might even make it to the hairdressers once the kids are back at school. But I need to find the money for the hairdressers. If I could just make some money, that would sort out all my problems.

12:28 pm: A secret: the first time Peter and I had sex, I got pregnant. Complete accident, just so drunk we forgot to use a condom. (Have I mentioned the sex was great?) We didn't see each other for a bit, just circumstances, then he explained that he was engaged. He was really sorry. I should have told him that I was pregnant, but I just couldn't do it. If I'd told him, he would have done the right thing and left college and got a job. And we would've ended up hating each other. So I planned an abortion, and made it all go away. He looked at me every time I entered a room. I couldn't show him how I felt, couldn't touch him in public, couldn't talk to him. It was awful.

12:33 pm: Sex is so much more exciting when you're young. Once you've given birth, having strangers touch you is not such a taboo, or such a novelty. We're like cows with vets reaching up us.

12:38 pm: Of course, sex can also be very embarrassing when you're young. I remember leaving a bar with two Spanish guys. I was a bit drunk, wearing a rather revealing dress that had hooks and eyes all down the front. That dress got me into so much trouble. The good-looking one said goodnight. I was so disappointed, I thought I was going to get both that night! In the not-so-good-looking guy's place, there was no furniture. Just a bare mattress on the floor. We had sex on the bare mattress. I lay there shivering afterwards and he leaned over and breathed into my ear, 'That was good, I make you have orgasms for me, yes?' And I replied: 'Orgasms! I'm effing freezing!'

1:00 pm: My partner is at a restaurant lunch with another woman today. Other women really like him. They say he listens! It would be nice if he'd go out to lunch with me. His office is only 15 minutes away. On second thought, he'd probably shout.

9:16 am: I've always wanted to have sex with the right man and multiple female partners. I would have to have a man who excites me. I love the feel of a man's body taking me, preferably from behind with me on all fours. But I would love to explore my attraction to women as well. To enjoy another woman's body, her soft vulva, wet and excited, moaning with pleasure beneath me as I take her like a man, maybe using a dildo. I get horny just thinking about it. But I would have to find the right, sexy man, and the right group of women willing to experiment and enjoy each other. I don't live in that world, though. And I'm just not attractive enough any more to play games like that. It will always remain a fantasy.

10:45 pm: I'm going to make this my last entry. I wish I'd known that Peter is the love of my life years ago. So often our fun phone sex ended with discussions of what might be, if only we could find a way to be together. We say we didn't want our partners to get hurt, but really we just didn't have the courage to change our lives. We'll probably end up in the same retirement home, too old and demented to recognise each other and I'll wonder why I want to kiss him so badly, this strange man in the plastic-covered seat across the room.

—⁓—

the unemployed dad-of-three with many exes, considering shacking up with his girlfriend

46, MALE, EDINBURGH

MONDAY

6:45 am: My girlfriend, who I haven't seen in a week, called and woke me up. She has a distinctive name, so I'm just going to call her Zena. Zena was wide awake. Something about us meeting up later today. Back to sleep.

10:37 am: Zena has just called me, wondering why I called her at 7:25. Difficult, since I was asleep! We have a lot of communication problems on the phone.

10:50 am: Zena has called again, inviting me to a picnic. I now have to decide between doing what I had planned to do today, and a picnic. I feel confused.

11:20 am: Decided on picnic, and am now in Zena's car. Spoke to her about her driving like a racing driver around built-up streets. She is unusually receptive today, and slowed down.

11:55 am: Sitting in the park in the sunshine, catching up on her life and mine and my three kids. It feels great.

2:00 pm: The conversation is serious now. We're talking about moving in together. We've been in-and-out of our relationship for five years. During that time we have both seen other people and continued our affair. In the last six months, we've worked at having a proper relationship. The main issue is that we both like our own space, which is difficult if we're living in the same place. That, and issues of trust and communication, though if we did live together, it would solve most of them.

3:10 pm: We lay down in each other's arms for an hour's sleep. Now she's just awoke, and decided that we're not going to live together. I'm frustrated that we're both out of work and can't move on and buy a house together.

4:00 pm: Lying together, looking at patterns in the clouds. After some discussion, the move is back on. I feel elated.

6:55 pm: Fish and chips at her place. Sometimes in a relationship you need someone who can kick you up the backside, like Zena. Every so often I need a dose of reality.

8:05 pm: Zena is having a cigarette. Serious foreplay was in process, kissing and touching each other intimately, until Zena decided she wanted to stop for a smoke.

8:35 pm: In bed making love. As usual, it is fabulous when it goes well.

10:15 pm: Zena's asleep with the TV on. I've just tucked her into bed, and will eventually fall asleep next to her.

TUESDAY

9:15 am: Awake at Zena's apartment. She just made me a cup of tea. This is her way of saying, 'Get up and go home, I have things to do.' Which suits me, as I have things to do too.

9:35 am: She's complaining about the way she looks. I am telling her she is gorgeous.

9:45 am: Dressed, big hug goodbye.

2:00 pm: On my way to an appointment, I am realising how happy I am in my current relationship. How do I know? I am not admiring every pretty girl who passes by. I can't really quantify what I like about Zena; I've just always been attracted, like moth to flame.

4:00 pm: Off to buy a birthday present for my young daughter. I have a very unpleasant relationship with her mother. I have tried to improve it, but she will not budge. My daughter hardly knows me, and every effort I make to change this is refused. I'm not sure if I should just give up and wait until she is older? Thinking about it makes me depressed.

4:30 pm: I've just run into my ex-wife's mother (my daughter's grandmother) in the shop. She doesn't recognise me. This may be a good thing.

7:00 pm: All the birthday shopping is done. Thinking about my daughter makes me depressed. I met her mother via Match.com while splitting from my first wife. We were a perfect match: I needed a home, she needed help paying the bills. We met Friday, I moved in Sunday. Life was great, until we had fertility treatments. That same week I met Zena, and I suddenly realised that I had met my ideal partner. It was like being hit over the head with a brick.

8:28 pm: Just had my beloved Zena on the phone. It's a little late for her to invite me to hers, so we've agreed to a quiet night alone. That's okay, as I want to talk to my adult son tonight and get up early.

10:15 pm: Spoke to my son Scott, and arranged to meet him Thursday. His mother and I are still friends, and have done some volunteer work together – I took that as a sign that although our relationship went down the pan, she still trusts me. We were together 15 years, and she left me for someone else – she probably beat me by a week.

2:25 am: Composing a huge long email to my daughter's mum complaining about my lack of access, despite the Child Support Agency quite happily taking hundreds of pounds per month from me. Her reasons change every time. Not happy. Zena and I are too old to have our own kids. I think my daughter is being cheated by her mother's stubbornness.

WEDNESDAY

12:49 pm: A late start today, not much to get up for. Have I mentioned that I'm unemployed?

3:00 pm: Was concentrating so hard on getting my daughter's present wrapped up for posting that I sent it off without signing her card. Must get another one.

4:00 pm: Looking forward to taking Zena to see my friend's band tonight. I must admit to being jealous of him: he has an attractive girlfriend who is supportive, and they seem very settled and content.

5:05 pm: Zena just called to say she is too busy to go out tonight. I am very disappointed. I could go round to see her, but we spend too much time sitting round talking about our relationship and not enough time having fun.

7:04 pm: Friend rang. His girlfriend died two weeks ago. He's sounding much better. I'm quite relieved that he's starting to look ahead.

9:30 pm: Watching my friend Luigi's band. They sound great, and there must be all of 20 people in the place.

10:15 pm: Gig over, and just called Zena as promised. She invited me round. I think she's had a couple of drinks, as she was slurring. I said I'd call her from home and maybe head up to her place with a bottle of wine.

10:35 pm: Zena can't remember why I am calling her. A couple of large vodkas were definitely involved. We egg each other on for a while to keep drinking. I'd love to see her, but I know we'll stay up late drinking, and she won't be in a fit state to drive the car in the morning.

10:37 pm: It's not like me to be so unselfish. Perhaps I am finally growing up?

1:00 am: It's late at night and I miss my girlfriend. I'm about to go to bed, and want to have a fantasy to masturbate over, so I'm looking for some porn on the Internet. Lots to chose from, but it's not really doing anything for me. I can see that it's all staged.

1:15 am: I found some Internet porn that turned me on: some guy having sex with some Asian-looking girl. What I liked about it was:
- I'm better looking than the guy
- My thing is bigger than his thing

Although at the end he came all over her face. I don't understand. Five billion years of evolution has programmed me to ejaculate *inside* somebody. Anyway, the bits before that part did make me feel quite excited.

THURSDAY

8:00 am: Off to a job interview and exam.

11:25 am: Tests completed. Very hard, but my forward planning seems to have paid off. I was the only person to finish, so I'm feeling quite smug.

1:30 pm: Sitting in the sun having a beer with my son. It doesn't get much better than this.

4:00 pm: Several beers later and a lecture in economics and politics from a 20-something. I am so proud. Starting to wonder if we brought the wrong baby home from the hospital.

7:30 pm: Lovely call from Kara. Three years ago we met on the Internet as friends. It soon became sexual and I was mostly very happy about it. We had one argument in six months. Fantastic sex and lots of love bites, with which I had great fun going into work and trying to cover up. Then Zena came back into my life. I really like her but I know she's not the one to spend my life with.

10:07 pm: Because of her mother's intransigence, I have missed my daughter's birthday. I did, however, get an email *almost* thanking me for the present.

11:08 pm: Zena has a friend staying. I know him well, and I know there is no sexual attraction between them. But I still feel left out. A simple phone call for 30 seconds would help significantly. And so will living together.

11:10 pm: You'll have to excuse me. It's not easy to type while tearing your hair out at the same time.

FRIDAY

6:00 am: Zena phones me at six in the morning, again. Zena! Why call someone at that time and not leave a message?

11:30 am: Having a jam session with two friends.

2:15 pm: Zena called twice during the practice, but I couldn't hear as it was way too noisy. She left a message asking why I didn't call her back. And then when I did call back, no answer!

4:03 pm: Zena called, and is not happy. We've both been waiting all day for each other to call. This happens a lot because she gets involved in things, promises to call back, and then forgets. Mobile phones mean that we are permanently in touch, but it does make things a bit intensive.

4:50 pm: Was just offered a job. This feels like a load lifted off my shoulders. Brilliant.

6:14 pm: Telling Zena the good news. She sounds much better. We agree to go for a drive tomorrow. I am pleased about this because we spend too much time indoors, navel-gazing and talking round in circles: we both complain about unemployment, then we quiz each other on past relationships, despite the fact that neither of us wants to talk about them.

7:07 pm: Now we're speaking about buying some land and building a house. It makes me feel very positive.

7:30 pm: Zena keeps calling me! She is very tired and really needs to get some sleep. I have only seen her once this week, and feel that she's making very little effort, with maximum annoyance. Fed up. I'm turning my phone off.

12:03 am: Zena's left a message saying that if I don't call back immediately, our day out tomorrow is cancelled. But my phone was off, so I didn't get the message until now. I was very happy with my relationship, but now I wonder if I really need the hassle.

—⁓—

the nurse with a baby, teenager and long-term partner, who is just fine without a marriage certificate, thank you

41, FEMALE, GLASGOW

THURSDAY

6:30 am: Am hoping David will continue where we left off yesterday morning, until the baby turned her early-morning baby babble into plaintive wailing.

6:42 am: The baby has curtailed against any encore of a sexual nature. David got up with her and I will have a lie-in.

8:35 am: I've dispatched the baby to nursery, and David has gone back to bed. The teenager, Libby is still in bed. We won't see her till lunchtime. I am going into work for a training that I was hoping was cancelled. Will have to leave a 'to do' list for David and Libby.

1:04 pm: Back home to find David doing his best to tidy things, with Libby. They get on fantastically. She says he is more a dad to her than her own dad. I dated David for six months before I introduced them.

1:55 pm: David is reminding me that I am on a healthy-eating kick. I now have a Victoria sponge instead of a muffin top around my midriff. He is super fit, and has been dragging me out running with him. I will always be slightly overweight, and when we have sex and it is daylight, I try to 'arrange' myself so that my tummy flab doesn't wobble. I wish I were much slimmer, but when we are having sex, I am the most ravishing woman in the world…

3:57 pm: Back from smear test. The practice nurse asked me about contraception. I told her that David and I are using condoms, because the baby was conceived after pill failure – my periods trailed off and I thought I was menopausal! David is now paranoid that it might happen again. Kind of ruins the post-coital warm haze moment when I see David standing by the side of the bed, knotted condom in hand, saying, 'Hah! Got you little bastards! No more surprises!'

3:59 pm: That, and when I squeeze my pelvic floors so hard when he is inside me that the condom comes off mid-thrust and he has to fish it out… We laugh about it.

4:00 pm: Libby is out. Hmm. I think she has a secret. She has been going out to 'clear her head' too often.

10:24 pm: Time for bed. Well, me anyway. We watched 'Bloomin' Hestontal' (our joke name for Heston Blumenthal) and *Spooks*, and now David is playing his online game. I won't see him till 2 am. Sometimes I really hate the game. However, I am lucky: David is not a womaniser or a drinker. Or a golfer. He is at home, being a complete geek. At 2 am he will snuggle up against me and nuzzle his face into the back of my neck, and we will sleep spooning. We are almost telepathic sometimes.

3:56 am: The baby woke up during the night and David sorted her out with a fresh nappy, milk and a cuddle.

FRIDAY

6:56 am: David's first question to me today: 'When are we going running?' Too busy today.

9:00 am: My girlfriends and their toddlers are round for tea and coffee cake. One asked why, after five years, we are not married. David and I started as friends. There was no instant falling in love, as he was in lust with someone else. We just kind of grew on each other, and I think that is why we have the kind of relationship we have now. No mad outpourings of undying love. We know we love each other without saying it – it is the little things. We are happily unmarried. And not-married is just the way we like it!

1:21 pm: David is cooking lentil soup for lunch. This morning Libby dressed the baby in a ridiculous outfit and I told her to change it. She hasn't spoken to me since.

5:00 pm: My old friend and colleague Mona is staying the weekend. She has filled me in on her disastrous relationship. Disastrous because they are still living in the same house, as they cannot sell it. We have had too many glasses of wine. She is outside having a ciggie.

8:23 pm: Oh my God, the kitchen! David has been cooking *all* day, and has used every pot, pan and utensil. All for a pork chop, potato dumping and a sponge cake. I don't dare tell him that I am still hungry. I just told him that the place looks like it was hit by a bomb. He's getting really defensive.

9:00 pm: Telling Mona about a letter I received from my ex: I had many small, insignificant relationships after my ex-husband and before David. One was a guy who I knew was to have an arranged marriage. It was quite intense, cramming as much time in together as we could in a year. I knew he wouldn't go against his parents' wishes, and I wouldn't allow him to meet Libby. Anyway, he is married now, and apparently unhappy. Our relationship meant something to me at the time, but in hindsight, it was nothing compared to what I have now.

9:59 pm: Discovered I unintentionally locked Mona smoking in the garden! She is bedding down for the night on the sofa bed, and Libby is in her room. I feel frizzy and am not sure why. Bedtime.

SATURDAY

7:30 am: Heard the baby and her babble through the monitor, and brought her to our bedroom. Libby came to the door soon after and took her downstairs to have breakfast with Mona. Trying to snuggle into David, but we are both distracted by the noise.

10:30 am: Went to have my hair cut for the second time in two weeks. Long story, but it involved being unfaithful to my hairdresser of ten years. I booked Mona in for a beauty treatment, and she feels well chilled now.

1:30 pm: Domestic bliss! David out at the town pool with the baby. Upstairs Libby is studying, and Mona and I are in the lounge drinking tea and reading the newspapers.

1:45 pm: I spoke too soon. Libby is in a strop because her 'bezzie mate' called to ask if she wanted to go shopping. I told her no, as we have visitors. I find it really hard not to rise to these teenage tantrums. Though we are lucky, as plenty of kids are out doing and drugs and having sex.

4:04 pm: I never imagined I'd be doing the suburban coupley cosiness. It was just me and Libby for all those years. My previous relationship ended when my ex-husband hit me. Libby was little, and I left. I had seen too much of that through work, and knew not to buy his 'but I love you' line. I waited a long time for someone like David to come along.

7:15 pm: Girly chat with Mona. We are out at a small restaurant that is one of David's favourite places, so it's a bit weird without him. He is staying home to babysit.

11:19 pm: Had a lovely meal out. We reminisced about relationships and gossiped about people we still know from those days. Fantastic meal.

11:23 pm: In bed now. David hasn't played his online game all evening due to a technical hitch. This happens every time he has a 'free evening' to play for as long as he likes. Told him that I had nothing to do with it. He laughed. I feel quite horny, hoping that he is up for sex.

11:45 am: David fell asleep. So no sex.

SUNDAY

8:37 am: About to go downstairs and get breakfast for everyone. Libby left me a note on my pillow, continuing the strop.

12:50 pm: Mona just left for her journey home. Feel quite a sense of loneliness – it was nice having her here. David is out training. The baby is refusing to have a nap. Spoke to Libby. She gave me that teenage 'get off my case' look.

5:46 pm: Back to work tomorrow, and I suddenly feel very overwhelmed with the things I have to do. I need to prepare and do some reading for work, and I feel so knackered. David wants to go for a run tonight. Even though it would be 15 minutes of exclusive time with David, the thought of donning a T-shirt that does nothing to flatter my bulky tum doesn't appeal. I am not sure he realises how tiring it is to do housework, run after a toddler, etc. Sometimes I feel really resentful, not towards him but just the situation. I don't get me-time to sit and write or read. And I only work part time!

5:56 pm: David is upstairs bathing the baby. I can hear her squeal over the funny things her daddy does. He is such a good man. Maybe I should just expose myself to teenage wrath by asking Libby to do more round the house.

6:01 pm: Cat wants in.

6:01 pm: Cat wants out.

6:01 pm: Cat wants in.

6:01 pm: Cat wants out.

6:02 pm: It is Libby's cat.

7:03 pm: Watching *Lost and Found* with the baby, 'ooooh' and 'ahhhhhh' being her vocabulary throughout the 50 minutes. Now her bedtime.

7:17 pm: I'm half hoping David has forgotten the run, and we can just have something to eat. I am feeling very hungry. Had cheese on toast at lunchtime. Nothing substantial. Going to tidy the baby's toys now and fetch the washing…

8:45 pm: Just finished a run, and in such a foul mood. Eating, finally.

11:00 pm: Watching crap TV, and now going to bed. No, diary, there was no sex! We have a great sex life, normally once or twice a week. I am lucky that in our entire relationship, we have never gone more than four weeks without having sex, and that was immediately before the baby's birth, and the three weeks after.

MONDAY

6:54 am: Been up since 6 am. So far, emptied the dishwasher, fed cats, mopped floor, mucked out the cat tray, packed the baby's nursery lunch, awoke the baby, changed and dressed her, dressed myself. Hopefully will brush my teeth. That's the bit that usually gets neglected, I'm ashamed to say.

6:17 pm: Very busy day at work – I had presentations to deliver. Libby in a strop over exams, the baby hyper after a day in nursery, David is doing techy geeky stuff. How come everyone else just goes off and does their own thing, and I am left with the domestic drudgery?

6:21 pm: David wants to go out for another run tonight. If the baby is not in bed, then I will not be going.

8:00 pm: Went out for a run. Actually enjoyed it, but I'd never tell David that. Size 8, here I come!

8:20 pm: Scuppered that dream by scoffing down a plate of chicken and rice, followed by ice cream sprinkled with chocolate.

9:05 pm: Bedtime now, very tired.

TUESDAY

6:30 am: Trying to think positive thoughts, like 'Doing this domestic drudgery is great because it means I have a roof over my head, and the mess is made by my beloved family and many people don't have these things.'

6:32 am: Feeling cheesed off because I am the one who cops the workload, and no one helps unless I repeatedly ask.

7:59 am: Back in bed. David is taking the baby to nursery, so I've made a cup of tea and asked him to bring a newspaper home, which I will read in bed before I start the day's to-do list.

1:44 pm: Being extremely lazy. Considering doing some work, but cannot muster the energy.

3:59 pm: Libby just in from school. She seems to be in a good mood, and thinks she did all right on exams. I have done absolutely nothing brain-stimulating today. David is collecting the baby, then out to play five-a-side tonight with the lads. They are the other halves of my friends. We all met through our babies.

7:52 pm: Libby is on the phone to her father. He's remarried. I haven't had contact with him for a long, long time. Libby is old enough now to make her own arrangements with him, and they must be getting on again. I am not required as go-between. Makes my life so very much simpler.

9:09 pm: Sending a text to my baby friends. We are all on our own, as our partners are all out playing five-a-side. Text came back asking me round for coffee when I'm off work Thursday. Cool.

9:52 pm: Going to sleep now. David not home yet. If I am asleep when he gets in, he will climb into bed behind me and put his cold hands on my boobs and snuggle up. This relationship is nothing like any I have experienced.

WEDNESDAY

5:15 am: Awake, cursing the lightweight curtains. David is spooned round me. I love feeling so encased and wrapped up in his arms. Our relationship is solid, safe, respectful, loving. With a good measure of passion thrown in.

6:17 am: The baby up and in a contented mood. She is sitting on my lap drinking her milk while I type.

9:59 am: Seemed ages to get to work this morning. Had to drop David off outside city centre, then double back. We hardly ever argue – only over driving and maps.

12:54 pm: Texted David to apologise for being grumpy for having to take him past his usual drop-off point. Not usually so snappy. Coming up for a week since we last had sex! Maybe that is the reason why.

3:30 pm: Collected the baby. I am out to Sainsbury's.

3:49 pm: Just got home. Libby and her friend are buzzing about their exams. Not that they would ask how my day has gone, but I had a really good day at work. I love doing trainings.

6:09 pm: David home, told me I am looking lovely. Maybe he is feeling the strain too. Tonight might be our lucky night!

7:15 pm: Libby and I had a big row over her spending £20 on her friend. Twenty! Her father gives her allowance, but gives me a big fat zero.

8:18 pm: Libby and I rowed again. She asked me what I do all day when I am at home! I snapped her face off.

8:23 pm: We made up. Having an evening of brain-numbing TV and a bowl of ice cream.

11:30 pm: Time for bed. David is playing online. Going to end here.

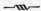

7

RELATIONSHIP
AS A LIFESTYLE

the sub dating a first-time dom with self-esteem issues

30, FEMALE, MANCHESTER

THURSDAY

8:01 am: Woke thinking of K. Masturbated to a complex Dominant/submissive scene (kneeling, bound, gag, plastic clothes pegs, riding crop and one very happy sub), an account of which i'm going to email Him to him in a minute – that's His current instruction for me. Even though all these things seem weird, i just love it. That's been a surprise for me: stuff i previously didn't even consider liking is now mind-blowing.

8:03 am: Note: i am writing of myself in lower case, and K in upper case, as a way of mentally reinforcing Dominance/submission status. This is very common in the D/s lexicon. Plus it's sexy. i never thought that just the act of writing in a submissive way would be sexy, but it bloody is.

9:21 am: K and i met on a BDSM website three months ago. He's an inexperienced Dom, and I've only been a sub once before. It's bloody brilliant. i find it hard to leave him. i really enjoy His idiosyncrasies, and because of the nature of the relationship, we have to be much more matched in terms of interests. Thanks, Internet, you're the best.

9:23 am: Some background for you: D/s relationships are a consensual exchange of power between a Dom (or Domme, aka Master, Top, Sir) and His or Her submissive (aka sub, slave boy/girl, bottom). It is commonly said that the bottom has the power over the Dom, because each time a sub chooses to submit, he or she has the option to say 'no', thereby deciding the Dom's authority. It's a negotiated dynamic.

9:35 am: On the phone with K. It's hard to be a newbie Dom. He's got lots of confidence issues from past relationships. He's going through the emotions of accepting that He wants to hurt someone He cares about. He's talking about how difficult it can be to go from loving and caring K, to Master. K and i are constantly discussing the ins and outs of the D/s scene, deconstructing our sessions together, and helping each other with the emotional bit. It's much more openly self-analytical than 'vanilla' relationships.

1:15 pm: Meeting K for lunch! Thai. He picked my lunch for me. So sexy!

1:48 pm: We just walked past His boss on the street. He's quiet and studious at work, and i know He gets a really big kick out of the fact that people have no idea what He's *really* like.

3:07 pm: At home, applying for education jobs, and rereading an email from W. Five years ago we had a short, intense Master/slave relationship which consumed me, because i was very inexperienced – i didn't even know i was a sub. Obeying him was like cracking open my soul. It was like he held me up to a mirror, and there i was. i'd been found. The discovery of this new thing made me drop everything and let myself just freefall. He was everywhere for me, and did what no one had ever done: he denied me, he moved me, controlled me, challenged me, seduced me. It was breath-taking.

3:09 pm: Different, though, than my current relationship. Master/slave is also consensual, but once committed, there was no option for 'no'. i was owned and 'collared', and signed a 'contract' establishing boundaries and terms. For me it was incredibly powerful to sign myself away like that. i do miss that unique feeling of (dangerously) handing my life over to him. i'd love to do a contract with K, but we are both finding our feet.

6:07 pm: K just called, apologising about being preoccupied at lunch (i didn't mind). He's taking the night off and asked if i want to come over. Fuck yeah.

6:40 pm: K just sent a text as Master: *You shall wear the balls tonight, you are aware of Master's presence even in His absence. Confirmation of insertion required.*

6:59 pm*: They shall remain in place until Master instructs otherwise.* Done.

9:30 pm: Didn't go over to see K, due to other plans i'd made with my housemate. Our main challenge is handling the shift between BDSM and normal stuff, like housemates. It's a bit weird sometimes. i have a few friends who are aware that i have slightly different interests, but no one really knows. i don't have any BDSM friends. In many ways that makes us even more dependent and locked into each other, as no one else would really get it.

9:35 pm: The balls make me think of W. The way i take instructions from K is completely different. i don't usually compare them, but i let W right inside, and i know that i block K on certain levels. Where W took me, i want K to take me further. But W also left me alone. i was just working out who i was – a strong, independent woman suddenly becoming someone else's slave – and he didn't reassure me.

10:01 pm: You'd probably want W to fuck you. He's very powerful. You would. i wanted it very much. But he knew that to deny the submissive sex gave him enormous power. i was insatiable. All i thought about was him. i couldn't function. We were together for six months, and he never fucked me. (Any boys reading this – denying women sex can have quite a powerful effect. Few men realise, as they're always trying to get laid. Hopeless.)

10:53 pm: Text from Master: *The balls may come out at the next convenient opportunity. To be pulled slowly and deliberately as they leave slave girl's slut body. Master is retiring for the evening. Goodnight.*

12:15 am: i'm going to bed. i'll probably think of K, and how much i enjoy seeing the Master that emerges from him. i may just call him ☺. We've spent the past few times together being loving and making love. i had been worried that just doing the BDSM side of play, and face fucking me (which He *loves*. Fucker. What am i saying? i love it too), would end up making our relationship hollow. He agreed. It's been wonderful. And following recent tenderness, we're moving back into Master/slave girl territory. i imagine that these are two states our relationship will flit between.

FRIDAY

9:28 am: Slept in, and off to do some volunteer work.

9:39 am: As if K has read my mind, He's suddenly in Master mode: *As previously instructed slave girl shall wear the balls while volunteering and shall notify Master promptly if she reads the news in that state.*

9:41 am: My response: *She did not bring the balls with her today. She apologises to Master.*

9:45 am: *That is most regrettable indeed, nor should she presume to refer to herself in upper case. Master is displeased.*

9:48 am: Me: *Master being displeased is very sexy.*

1:15 pm: Just spoke to K. He's been feeling very Dom all day. i love it. When He's in Master mode and being instructive and hard to please, i go very into my happy sub-world.

1:23 pm: On Sunday i went into pretty deep 'subspace' for the first time, and He's keen to get me into that state again. Subspace: The physiological and psychological descent from total consciousness to the relaxing, uninhibited plane of submission. i'd known of it, but didn't know what it actually was until Sunday. It was mind-expanding. K has achieved what W never did.

1:29 pm: Sunday was an extended session using pegs and nipple clamps on my breasts. i should say that D/s takes on many form, so everything is 'sex', with or without penetration. K has a plan, though often it just starts up. i will ask for K to do things like slap me, or He will just decide. He finally removed the clamps, after tormenting me for a while, and i suddenly became incredibly submissive, but also very tired, and curled up against Him. i thought i'd fall asleep, but suddenly i was so unbelievably submissive and my mind in a completely different universe. It is an incredible high, like ecstasy. He could have done anything He pleased. It was incredible. It's like your body and your mind are both separated but also connected to every molecule in the air.

4:00 pm: One of the volunteers just noticed a dirty mark on my face and tried to clean it off. It's a small bruise. She laughed and joked, 'Is your new man hitting you?'

4:03 pm: i just found out that i like being slapped across the face. It's all about headspace, really. Slapping me when we are in a scene is amazing. Slapping me when we're more in vanilla mode is awful, just awful. Last week i was feeling submissive and happy, and He made me go down on Him, and then began slapping my face. i just burst into tears. He comforted me and we talked about it. i think He is more aware of the signs that i would like to be slapped. That's why communication and understanding is a billion times more essential here than in vanilla relationships.

8:00 pm: Call from my mum. She's the love of my life, if it's okay to describe a non-sexual partner that way. She supersedes and transcends everyone.

9:45 pm: K and i just spoke. It seems funny to slip from a Dom day, back into normal K and me mode. It reminds me of a moment with K a few weeks ago when i was on the bed, bound and deprived of my senses (blindfold, gag, ear plugs). Anyway, K just suddenly stopped, and i knew He had stopped. He left the scene and came back a few minutes later to untie me, and we talked about it. He said that just for a moment, He had seen the level of control He had, and the darkness inside it. To most people that would seem possibly frightening, but there was something about it, that He was as exposed as i was, naked and underneath Him. It was quite beautiful.

9:57 pm: Why do i have a desire to be harmed? my submission is about not hiding the parts of myself that i don't like. Not just from my partner, but from myself. Suffering is an incredibly strong compulsion; i fantasise about being made to cry. my immense desire to be harmed, abused, humiliated was one of the things i took a long time to accept about myself. i'm now of the opinion: i have no idea why i like it, but i do. What's more difficult to explain is consenting to things i don't care for. For example, i fucking hate being whipped with a cane or a riding crop (flogged). It hurts, i don't connect with it. He enjoys it. i consent to that. Then there are my hard limits. They are: tickling, blood, needles, scat, knives and public or outdoor play. He respects that and He'd never do it. But He enjoys hearing my pain/discomfort. Not the 'pain' itself, but having Him witness my pain. If you can get your head around that, then let me know.

SATURDAY

11:14 am: Morning K text: *K has a raging hangover horn and needs a good sucking.*

11:15 am: Part of me wants to drive right over. i hope He continues today. i like it when He's stern and grouchy and displeased. i love to please Him, and being told i'm a good girl. But He often lets me have what i need too easily as a Master. In a session if i beg to orgasm, He lets me. Deny me, for the love of God. He has a lot to learn.

11:17 am: Maybe he's missing that a thing i like about my submission is shame. My guess is that most subs are driven by either pain or humiliation. i like the latter far, far more than pain. Pain is easy to administer and, i suppose, process. Humiliation is different. He's asked me to detail my fantasies, but those around humiliation are hard to express. Example: say you have a huge fantasy to lick a toilet seat (i don't), and your Dom forces you to ask to do it. The shame you feel to confess it is as humiliating as the act. It puts you into amazing headspace.

12:15 pm: Remembering talking online to a Dom who seemed interesting. Then he asked if i was into 'K9'. He said it was being fucked by a dog. Christ – HARD LIMIT! It's amazing how weirdly normal it is to discuss these extremes, though, even meeting in real life. ('Oh you like enemas too. Great!')

4:21 pm: Going to enjoy a bit of sun now. i'm looking forward to seeing K tomorrow for two whole days of us.

7:00 pm: Don't feel well, went to bed, and found myself lying there thinking about Him.

9:57 pm: Just texted K. He's coming to pick me up and take me to His. i had this immense urge to be with Him.

11:30 pm: He came and picked me up, i was so happy. i could've driven over, but He likes to pick me up and it's lovely. He looked after me and He held me when i needed. i felt so much better – i think we both did. When we are together, life makes more sense.

1:15 am: We made love, and it was glorious. There's something about just being in the missionary position, with my arms around him, eye contact, kissing and touching in a different way. It's lovely.

2:15 am: We talked some more. Now i am back in submissive mode via His manipulation of my nipples and me licking His cock. (When i'm submissive, i lick things.) Spectacular. Eventually we'll sleep.

SUNDAY

10:03 am: i love waking up next to K.

12:09 pm: i'm woken up feeling very submissive, and began with cock worship, indulging in pleasuring His cock for a long time, though it's not entirely just a blow job. K spent a long time fucking my mouth and making me gag. Eventually He came, and i was still feeling uber-subbie, so He began manipulating my nipples, which really sent me down into a dreamy, trance-like subspace. Especially when He clamped pegs on to them, as i lay across Him weak and dreamy. About a minute later He told me to get on the floor and guided me by my hair (hmmmm) into the bathroom.

12:24 pm: A digression here is around my thoughts on being pissed on. It's about being covered in it, and taking my headspace *low*. What did i like about it? Feeling degraded, knowing He was going to do it. Years ago i wasn't sure whether i actually wanted to do it, and drinking it was a definite no-no. My disappointment was that He left me in the bath for about 15 to 20 minutes in self-bondage (kneel, put your hands on the bath rails, don't move – subs will maintain their state of bondage without physical restraints). The trippy, blissfulness subsided a little bit. i knew K was downstairs drinking His body weight in water.

12:51 pm: Then He came back. He peed on me. A lot. Hair, skin. Everywhere. i have to say i can't believe how much i loved it. There, i said it. i even opened my mouth.

12:53 pm: Then He made me suck His cock. But by then i couldn't do any more. The pegs were beyond painful, i couldn't think. i gagged. i knew it'd take Him ages to orgasm again. It was quite obvious i was waning. i said i had to stop. We stopped. i begged Him to take the pegs off. He did, very quickly, and it felt like my nipples were being pulled off. (Clothes pegs numb nipples after several minutes. When the peg is removed, blood rushes back into the capillaries and pain is revived.) Christ.

12:59 pm: He crouched down and kissed me and asked if i was okay. i nodded. i said i couldn't do any more. He said i did really well. Then He turned on the shower to clean me. We showered together, we touched and cuddled in the shower. Then into the bedroom to deconstruct the scene. It was great, i kept saying that i couldn't believe how much i enjoyed it.

1:30 pm: i think it was then that i went all submissive and subspacey again as a delayed reaction to the removal of the pegs – there is a direct correlation between pegs on nipples, their removal and my subspace. i floated even more than before. And we had sex, more lovemaking, and i was in a different universe, and i could touch everything in the world and feel every emotion. There were clouds and my eyes kept fluttering closed and open and i'd see snatches of the universe and of K and i could feel every single eyelash. And we came and i just wanted to sleep and smile.

2:35 pm: Then i wanted to eat. That's all i was capable of doing. And drinking water.

3:54 pm: Then He ball-gagged me, gaffer-taped ankles and knees (i love gaffer tape), put cuffs on and tied my collar to the bed and left for 30 minutes to do work. Being bound-but-comfortable, say on a bed, and left alone, is so relaxing. i can't do anything but stay there. It just clears my mind.

4:20 pm: He came back and took off gag, fed me water. We talked for a while. i needed the loo, and He got me to edge/hop my way there with my knees still gaffed. Then i dozed off.

5:00 pm: Important: don't fall asleep while gagged and bound, because when you wake up you have no fucking idea what's going on and panic. Which is what i did. i could only breathe through my nose and my legs wouldn't move. i shouted, but K had music on next door and couldn't hear me. (He should ALWAYS be able to get to me if i need Him. BUT HE COULDN'T FUCKING HEAR ME. HUGE NO-NO.)

5:05 pm: Then i realised that although my wrists were bound and locked together, the buckles weren't, so i undid them, shouting for K. By this time K had heard me and came in. i was shouting, 'Get me out, get me out,' and crying. He was trying to calm me, i just wanted him to stop. i cut off the gaffer, stormed into the bathroom, pulled out the pleasure balls, threw them on floor, threw ball gag. Angry, angry, angry.

5:20 pm: Back in the bedroom, He said that He misjudged and was deep into His work. i was upset. It was His fuck-up. i was in His care. i told him if it goes wrong, it's down to Him to sort it out.

6:00 pm: We talked. It was okay. i put on make-up and we went to the park, walked around.

7:15 pm: K is cooking and i want to help Him. i feel wonderful, even though for the vast majority of the day we've been gloriously depraved together. Hurrah for BDSM. i am ravenous. Epic munchies.

9:22 pm: We're hanging out on the sofa talking about stuff, laughing with each other, watching funny things on YouTube, congratulating ourselves on how brilliantly perverted we are. Sleep soon.

MONDAY

11:15 am: We spent the morning lounging in bed talking, touching, smiling, eye contact, laughing about things nice and nasty. We decided it will be good to 'train' me to increase my pain tolerance to flogging, since it's an inevitable part of our play. i wonder if there's subspace potential there. Breakfast.

11:20 am: He just asked what else I'd like to do sexually. Sounds funny given the rest of this diary, but i've never had sex with a woman. i tend to go for men, but from time to time i'm really attracted to women. But i just wouldn't know where to begin – i know how men work, i don't know how women work, nor how i would approach one i like?

1:20 pm: K announced that He had a plan, and we began a scene. He bound my head in tape that only sticks to itself (not skin), like having a skin-tight rubbery mask on my head. It felt fantastic. He covered my mouth so i could breathe through my nose. He chained me on all fours, and tried pegs on my nipples, but the pain was excruciating from yesterday. He informed me He was going to use the riding crop and flog my arse ten times. i screamed into my gag, i could feel my eyes prickling with tears.

1:25 pm: It's horrible waiting to be struck by a cane or whip. i tense up and sweat but my palms prickle with anticipation, my heart speeds up and my breathing goes out of control. And He flogged me, and i screamed. Then it was over.

1:35 pm: He fucked me after that.

1:40 pm: We stopped when He had trouble getting me disconnected from the spreader bar. We lay on the bed together and talked. Previously we'd talked about how i wanted Him to be able to make me cry, and K had speculated that a key to that might be flogging.

3:00 pm: He is correct. K tried me again with the paddle. It really hurt, spanking over the existing welts on my arse, and i counted out loud, my voice quivering. He said it really aroused Him knowing that i was trying to cope with it.

3:08 pm: Then subspace kicked in – delayed reaction from the flogging. And my God was He beautifully, amazingly, spectacularly nasty. i was on my knees, prostrate on the bed sucking His cock as He pulled my hair and slapped me. Then He fucked me again, and this time i completely submitted my body – i was incapable of doing anything but kneeling. He man-handled me, slapped me, pulled my hair until He finally came, and pushed my face to the floor to mark the end of the session. i was so fulfilled, content, aroused and peaceful. He pulled me up by my hair and stared at me – this amazingly nasty expression on His face. Fucking incredible. i thanked my Master and He sent me off to clean. i was grinning from ear to ear. i came back and snuggled up to Him and let the greatness of that final session of the day seep in.

6:00 pm: We're making dinner. He thinks my excitement at jacket potatoes is cute.

8:00 pm: We went upstairs to talk, and sign up for a charity bike ride. i don't think either of us especially thought we'd have more sex. But lo, a little while later, i was licking Him all over His neck and back. Licking Him seems to only go one way, to D/s. It never leads to lovemaking.

TUESDAY

9:45 am: The side effects of being a sub kick in the next day when you wake up: blotchy skin on face from stubble and semen, bruises (knees, plus one on each ankle from the spreader bar), aches from maintaining a position for a long time, marks on my breasts and forearms from being grabbed, welts on my arse from the crop, very tender nipples from enthusiastic pegging. And hunger. So very, very hungry.

9:47 am: Thought: If only my ex could see me now. He's very conservative, and blindly religious, and believed that dancing and drinking would send people to hell. We lived together – in retrospect i realise we're both submissive.

9:49 am: Email from K:

> *Morning you, I hope you're well. I feel amazing. I have a warm glow*
> *circulating around my body from deep in my abdomen. I am truly in*
> *love. You are incredible. Can't wait to see you tomorrow.*
> *Have a great day,*
> *Your Master, lover and boyfriend.*

9:49 am: What a lovely message. i feel amazing, like we get to be ourselves, and that He'll come with me on whatever this adventure is. i don't just feel happy, i feel subspace. And that, boys and girls, is like joy crack.

9:50 am: i have no idea how K is able to work today.

10:15 am: Emailed K to tell Him about my masturbation fantasy this morning.

11:25 am: What an amazing 48 hours. He's just fucking wonderful. K said something that i thought was so beautiful: that He's doing this to someone He loves more than anyone He's ever loved. i can't remember what point He was making, because those words sounded so beautiful.

—〰—

the nudist lorry driver marrying his mistress

48, MALE, BERKSHIRE

FRIDAY

3:30 pm: Left the UK on Tuesday afternoon and have been on the road since then, dropping off loads and collecting my return load. I'm a removals man.

4:51 pm: Just stocked up with fish and bread and beer at the supermarket, and hope that a potential date for tonight works out – I think she'll bottle out, something to do with the husband.

5:15 pm: While driving towards our casa in Spain, mulling over K. I first came across K at a British Sunday morning market in Spain. She was wearing a white sexy dress and had an amazing figure, dress size 8, and her first words to me were to ask me if I was a stripper. God knows why she asked that, but I was butter. Since that day, me and my girl have visited her a few times and I've done some work for her. My girl's set me the challenge of pulling K! Life is so tough.

5:18 pm: K's got a great body but not a lot of grey matter. I hate to admit it, but it's just the body!

5:30 pm: My girl and I lived here full-time for a few years, great, but we did get a touch bored. The other Brits we met were very shallow with aimless lives. We moved back to the UK and it's good to be near the six kids again. Still waiting for text from potential date.

5:16 pm: Back in my casa, all is well here: no floods, fallen walls or nasty bugs. I think I'll grill the fish with olive oil, seasoning and frying peppers. Not heard from the potential date. Think she's going to blow out, and to be honest, the date would be good, but now I feel like chilling naked in front of a good movie.

6:12 pm: Emailing my girl back home. Wondering what she is doing, probably settling down to paint. I am engaged to a wonderful lady whom I love very much. We definitely have an open relationship. She is actively bi and I am straight – sometimes we share. We are practising nudists and we plan to marry this summer. We still have sex every day after 12 years.

9:22 pm: Home alone, no great surprise. Chatting to my lover via Yahoo chat. She's just given me a lecture on not chasing the girl this end hard enough. We are honest and don't have sex without telling each other.

9:30 pm: Am enjoying naughty thoughts, but really haven't got the energy.

10:04 pm: Enjoying the freedom of being naked after a soak in the spa tub. It was great to feel the bubbles massaging all over my naked body.

SATURDAY

7:15 am: Slept quite well, just Yahoo-ing my lover, she's got a day off today so I encouraged her to take her new car out for a spin. Need to wash some clothes and get them dry before heading off – I will have to be naked while I wash them, and it's not looking great weather-wise. There must be a setting for quick wash?

8:51 am: I'm in the driving seat till tomorrow lunchtime, torrential rain. I hope to pick up a hitch hiker – girl would be great, blow job amazing. Only happens in the pages of magazines.

9:29 am: Wash done. I hate putting my clothes on, but I guess I must. Time to hit the road, hoping to get as far as Burgos tonight.

2:53 pm: Just stopped for a coffee break and caffeine top-up. I'm just south of Madrid. Pretty uneventful journey so far. Many of my thoughts focus around women and sex – I'm trying to think mature, sensible thoughts, but they all end up the same way. I am addicted to sex, as is my partner, which is helpful.

3:27 pm: Pee, coffee and pancetta bocadillo. Been in my cab, chatting by Yahoo to my lover. Originally her husband was my lodger! He was such a prat, I couldn't believe how awesome his wife was. She eventually got rid of him and we set up a business together, and passions eventually took over.

3:40 pm: Still on Yahoo, my girl's talking to some friends we did a nude tour of Australia with. She's always outdoors and naked and uninhibited, preferably on a beach with palm trees! She's not helping my concentration. I've got a woman who needs sorting.

9:11 pm: At Borgos, fed and watered, calamari and beer. Now tucked up in my cab with the sound of rain. To be honest, evenings like this are tough and lonely. I'm bright but never really fulfilled my potential.

9:30 pm: Thinking about my kids, wish they'd tell me how they feel about the wedding. I get on really well with all but one – but they've never truly forgiven me for the affair that caused the marriage to break up. My marriage was fine. Me and my lover kept our affair quiet for four years, but there came a time eight years ago when I admitted it, and left my wife for my present lover. We've been together for 12 years now. I've said sorry to the kids, but it's tough for them.

9:32 pm: My wife was a naturist, and the children were brought up as naturists, but during their teens they were allowed to choose. They know we are nudists but don't participate with us. Feel real bad about being such a bastard because my wife didn't deserve it, but I fell in love and still am.

11:07 pm: Been chatting to my girl on webcam. Talked about how we're going to do art more seriously. Clothing was an option that we didn't go for, so I'm not sure how I concentrated on such a heavy subject. It's a good thing I've got curtains in my cab!

SUNDAY

6:13 am: 'Clothes are for special occasions,' says my lover. Today's special occasion is that it's bloody freezing. Still in sleeping bag, engine running and waiting for cab to heat up before I brave putting trousers on. Was at my proudest when I awoke.

6:20 am: I have an exciting laptop screensaver when I'm on the road. No, it's not pictures of my lovely kids. It's pictures of our nudist travels, fun, risqué and attached to brilliant memories. There's also photos of my lover with various girlfriends doing what she does well.

6:59 am: My girl's still sleeping, but left her an ushy message. For readers not in the know, 'ushy' is when you feel all filled up with lovey emotional feelings – it's a wonderful thing and it's okay for men to feel it.

2:15 pm: Boarding the ferry at Santander. Twenty-four hours of 'me' time now. Sitting in my cabin fiddling on my laptop. Looking forward to seeing my lover and catching up on our love life.

3:46 pm: Now sailing out. Did a strip for her to make her laugh. She laughed! Will shortly lose my signal.

MONDAY

1:11 pm: Just sailing into Portsmouth on a grey day. Spent most of my time in the cabin watching a couple of movies, and yes, a little porn. And yes I did – twice. The stuff I watch is usually run-of-the-mill heterosexual sex films or all girls. And my favourite is arty stuff. Not going to admit to watching anything else.

1:30 pm: Just wrote to my kids about the wedding, saying I love them, explaining a few things and asking what their honest thoughts are. Kids can be very straight-talking, gulp. My relationship with my boys is very 'matey'. My eldest is still hurting and has not forgiven me. I love her very much.

1:45 pm: Arranging for a naked dinner party in London next week. We've just got involved. We meet up and eat together naked. It all seems very proper, though, not exactly risqué. Things may change.

3:15 pm: While driving, thinking about my few bedroom regrets: Wish I had had more fun when younger. And I never slept with a coloured girl, which does appeal. And maybe I wonder what a cock feels like to touch. Not a conversation piece with friends. And I'd love to be in a porn movie or two. I did a couple a few years ago, and got paid. Loved it. Offers welcome.

5:26 pm: I'm home to the smell of roasting lamb! And a beautiful girlfriend who's made the effort and looks great. We've sat down and enjoyed a cup of tea and caught up. My girl's found a holiday she fancies in the Canaries that's open-minded nudist – looking forward.

6:39 pm: Lamb was awesome and clothes are starting to come off. There's nothing like feeling desired by your woman. I'm chilling with the telly.

6:40 pm: I jump every time I hear an email coming in on my BlackBerry. Not had any response to my mails to the kids earlier. The wait continues.

7:42 pm: Sat with my lover watching telly and discussing our swinging honeymoon. Waiting for a programme on Picasso before we head to the boudoir for romance and lovemaking which will probably turn into a good shag.

8:00 pm: Lover rabbiting on about wanting a kune kune pig. Not sure being on her own is good for her.

12:35 pm: All plans of romantic lovemaking went to pot as soon as we got our hands on each other's bodies. We just got filthy. First time she was on top, second time I was on top. A night of sex and passion was had.

TUESDAY

7:49 am: Woke this morning to her sitting astride and helping herself. Life is great! Now showered and breakfast cooking, and she's working. Today I'm off to Weston-super-Mare to deliver my load.

9:03 am: Emailing swinging nudist holiday place to say we're interested if the price is right. Also had mail from a couple. Don't get me wrong, we are not heavy swingers, and my girl is more keen on threesomes with another girl. We've enjoyed same-room fun with couples, and we have a couple of mates who she likes to strip for. Now she is asking more about swinging and the libertine movement, which I need educating on.

5:41 pm: Just got back from Weston-super-Mare; my girl should be home soon. I've got some spuds roasting in olive oil and paprika to go with lamb and some other things I've yet to decide on. Brownie points.

6:58 pm: Showering together and discussing the holidays. Considering a swinging place in Lanzarote, but it's new and we know nothing of the people running it. Think we'd prefer Cap D'age in France, where we love the beach and public shagging – there's nothing like the turn on of being watched.

8:15 pm: Just opened the mail. Credit card has taken a slamming. The engagement ring is worth every penny, it truly is. Rather than doing anything fancy, I took her to a favourite childhood haunt and asked her to marry me, and we just enjoyed each other's company.

9:30 pm: My girl's being a mum on the phone. Our kids are different, hers being quiet and boring, mine being outgoing and fun. We all get along, though.

9:30 pm: She just did a strip show, and we enjoyed some long, drawn-out sex, great as ever. To bed early.

WEDNESDAY

7:52 am: We got busy talking about fears in our relationship this morning and it just turned us on! In the meantime eggs are frying and breakfast served by naked woman is heading my way.

9:41 am: Here I am back at a ferry port, Portsmouth. This morning my lover asked me about any fears I have about our relationship. I couldn't think of any. There's nothing she could do to frighten me, not even intercourse with another guy. In fact, I'd love to watch. She's afraid I'll get bored. After 12 years, I'm not sure I will. She is awesome and I am besotted.

9:49 am: Heading for Barcelona. Unfortunately no time. There are free pole-dancing clubs along the seafront – I'd love to see my girl giving it a go. It's her secret desire as well. She says she would have been a stripper if we'd been together in our youth.

10:05 am: No crumpet spotted yet. One day I'll pull on a ferry and another fantasy will be fulfilled.

10:30 am: Could do with some naughty friends on Yahoo chat. Only person available is the girl who messed me around in Spain a few days ago. My girl says I should be persistent, but I can't be bothered. She's probably crap in bed anyway.

10:51 am: Just chatted to my best buddy online. He's really hot for my girl. For his private stag night she fed him champagne from her pussy. He'll always remember that one! It's his third wedding anniversary tomorrow to a fat bird. Yuck!

THURDAY

10:03 am: Coming into Santander on a hazy morning. Email from my lover about a secluded nudist retreat in Southern Mexico for our honeymoon. We'd be staying in a beach hut – how perfect can it be.

7:07 pm: Coming into Barcelona, honeymoon booked! Naked in Mexico.

7:51 pm: Just heard that three of my kids won't be attending the wedding. Feeling gutted and a bit emotional. Their mother is still single and they are being protective of her.

9:16 pm: Tucked up in my cab outside of Barcelona. Feeling a bit low, found today's drive exhausting.

9:30 pm: Need to find a smile, so I emailed for a girlfriend to come and stay with us in a couple of weeks. That'll mean threesomes and twosomes all round. She's a regular girlfriend we've known for years, and we all know what we want (sex). She's a decade younger than us, and I'm not really sure how it started, but we just got intimate, supported each other through tough times and now have a great relationship that works for all. How do I feel? Lucky.

—m—

the slave whose life is controlled by a queen he hardly knows

43, MALE, BIRMINGHAM

SATURDAY

4:45 am: Checking for an email from my Queen. Nothing! i think of my Queen and want to masturbate, but fear orgasming, so i will decline.

4:48 am: i am an owned slave. My Queen owns me and controls every aspect of my life. i am constantly in fear of failing her. As a slave, i am lower than all people, especially Mistresses. My insignificance is demonstrated by the small 'p' in my name, pansy, and small 'i'.

5:27 am: Couldn't sleep, so i masturbated. To ensure i did not climax, i dwelt on Jackie from HR. i imagined she was going to put me in to chastity.* My Queen allows others to use me for their benefit – tonight i'll be serving a Mistress and her two friends. They prohibit me from climaxing a week before they see me. This is normally to amuse themselves with my humiliation.

5:29 am: Updating my Queen with my schedule by email, as i have every day for three years. i fear her response. My Queen's words make me experience emotions at their extremity. A word of praise sends me on a euphoric high, but the suggestion that i have been slack in my work makes me feel like shit.

---

* An erotic device that prevents men from enjoying erections.

8:45 am: My Queen expects my work to be thorough: i am to keep this diary, and to research tickets for Paul McCartney. i do not believe Paul McCartney is to her taste, and as such, i fear there is an alternative motive.

12:15 pm: A text from Mistress A, telling me when and where i am to serve her and her friends.

3:00 pm: Driving to another city to serve Mistresses A, M and P this evening. Mistress A is a lady who wants to become a Mistress, who i met on a BDSM website. My Queen ordered me to do all to help her in her journey. Mistress P – let's call her Mistress Pain – is a pain mistress showing Mistress A the ropes, as it were. i have no say in this. To these Mistresses i am their sub (submissive); to my Queen, i am her slave.

6:30 pm: Arrived, chatting with Mistresses A and M. Mistress A has just told me that she'll be sure that Mistress Pain does not hurt me, as she is normally very sadistic. Her concern reassures me – i am not really into pain, but purely humiliation. Last time i served Mistress Pain, she said that i am a genuine sub/slave, and not a wannabe.

7:30 pm: The Mistresses asked me to photograph them in their outfits. i used to do photography, and my Queen has advised me that she now owns my skills for the benefit of others, to become an erotic photographer.

8:00 pm: Mistress Pain has arrived. This confuses me, as i was told that the games would start at 9 pm. i am introducing her to Mistress M, and working on making open conversations that they can all join in.

8:20 pm: Mistress Pain is showing me her nipple clamps. They are different from the others i have seen. My nipples are so sensitive. i fear that these monsters could make me fail my Queen and speak a safe word. My Queen has ordered me that i am not permitted to use any safe word. My own desires are of no significance. What is important is the desires of others. i exist to serve.

8:40 pm: The Mistresses have changed. Mistress A is in a basque and stockings; Mistress Pain a PVC dress and 'fuck me' heels; Mistress M in stockings and suspenders. All arouse me for different reasons: Mistress A's cleavage; Mistress Pain's heels; Mistress M's amazing legs.

8:45 pm: i am told what i must wear: PVC stockings and gloves. Otherwise completely naked. It is very humiliating. i am only five inches when erect, but lassie, the name my Queen has given my penis, has a tendency to shrink to an unbelievably small size. This said, after the beating, i will be oblivious to him.

8:50 pm: i just stroked lassie to get him to an acceptable size. Now i am sitting, awaiting the ladies to photograph them.

9:20 pm: Mistress Pain just tied my hands, and put two hoods over my face and tied it tightly round my neck. Annoyingly, they are pink cotton. i am blind, and she is tormenting my nipples with the clamps, making them hurt so much. i am shocked how the hood makes everything so much worse. Your mind takes over and alters the reality of what's occurring to you.

10:20 pm: i am kneeling over my knees with my hands on the sofa. They have just finished smacking me with their hands for what i assume was an hour, and whipping me with my own riding crop, continuously. Mistress M is an expert with the whip, and is teaching. The pain is a torment, and i cannot and do not understand how some people get off on it. The worse was when someone kept whipping my sensitive nipples with a riding crop. After some time i could not discern whether i was whipped with a ruler, riding crop or hand. i think they want to make me say the safe word.

10:50 pm: i am on all fours, and they have inserted anal beads. My bottom hole is very tight and i do not take any pleasure from this.

11:15 pm: They are playing a game. One person whips me, and i must guess who. If i am wrong, i am severely whipped five times. i have only got one right. i am also whipped across the shoulder if i cry out anything besides 'thank you'.

11:29 pm: i am wondering when Mistress M and Mistress A will save me. This is far more severe than i had considered. If i did not have my orders from my Queen to not say the safe word, i would have stopped well before now. But if i say the safe word, it means that my own comfort means more to me than my devotion to my Queen.

12:00 am: Mistress Pain: 'Everyone has their breaking point.' They are trying to break me.

12:05 am: They are taking a break, as their hands are tired. Mistress M: 'Oh my God, i think you are amazing. i never knew that this was so much fun! i am hooked.' So this is why no one has stopped. They have found this far more erotic than they anticipated.

12:20 am: If i move an iota, i will be punished. Never have i been so still. Mistress Pain is whispering into my ear: 'So, pansy, how close are we to your safe word?' Silence. 'Well, Mistresses, there is a part of his body that has no yet been played with. CBT, pansy, CBT.' i have no idea what this means.

12:21 am: Then it dawns on me: cock and ball torture. She is tying elastic cord so tightly around my balls.

12:30 am: Mistress Pain, whispering into my ear: 'pansy, if this makes you feel sick, you must tell me. i do not want you to bear it, you must tell me.' i feel tenderness towards her for saying this. She adds, 'Good, repeat what i have just said so that i know you understand?' i warm to her.

12:31 am: She just added sternly: 'For if you are sick in my hood, pansy, you will lick every drop up with your tongue.' The torturing has commenced.

1:30 am: Their games have ended. i have not spoken the safe word. i feel no sense of accomplishment – just fear that next time will be worse, and that i will not be able to hold out. Mistress Pain is leaving.

2:00 a.m: Mistress M and Mistress A are the best of friends. After much drinking, they are going to sleep in separate rooms. i am told that i will be going from bedroom to bedroom to serve them personally, as they see fit.

2:05 am: i first will go to Mistress M, and lick her out to make her orgasm many times.

3:00 am: i am back in Mistress M's room, as she then sent me to serve Mistress A, but Mistress A is on her period, so she sent me back to Mistress M. Again i am to lick her out and finger her until she comes.

4:30 am: i am back with Mistress A, who is now asleep, so i will sleep in her bed.

SUNDAY

2:00 pm: Spending the whole day with Mistress A and M. My bottom is sore whenever i sit down. But the pain is a distant memory, and they are pleased with me, congratulating me on taking so much pain, and i feel great pleasure in their pleasure.

2:10 pm: They are also letting me know that next time they will get the safe word out.

2:25 pm: Mistress M is asking about my previous service. My Queen, on one occasion when i annoyed her, made me serve a male Dom as punishment. i spent an evening with him at his home. i had to clean his bathroom, naked and collared. i had to suck his cock, then he bound and gagged me while he inserted many devices into my arse. i took little pleasure from any of this, but i do not have choices in such things. That is the whole point.

6:39 pm: Home. Just responded to a Fetlife casting call for a male nude model. i shall advise my Queen. i don't feel comfortable, but i must always serve wherever there is a need, regardless of whether it is sexual, BDSM or otherwise. i must gain permission only if it will interrupt my service of my Queen, or if it provides personal enjoyment. i have not followed football for two years now, despite being an avid fan.

8:36 pm: Emailed a full report of my weekend to my Queen. i am unclear whether she will be pleased with me or not.

9:06 pm: Email from my wife. We have been married for five years, and everyone assumes our relationship is wonderful, as we get on so well as friends. We separated eight weeks ago. i would be happier if she moved on, but her religious views prevent this from occurring.

9:15 pm: Considering how i can show her that the marriage is over. i have never told my wife of my Queen's ownership of me. i told her of my submissive desires, and confessed that i have served Mistresses, which she finds sick. She says that God can heal me, and that she will play a more dominant role in our marriage. i will not accept this, for these reasons:

1) My wife does not really want this. She is more submissive than dominant.

2) It would not satisfy me. My satisfaction comes from being to a Mistress what she craves.

3) BDSM should be 'safe, consensual and sane'. Anything else is a form of abuse. It is a very fine line. If my wife did this purely to keep our marriage, it would be a form of abuse.

10:10 pm: Completing many tasks for my Queen. i feel so tired yet must continue promoting her friend on Facebook, as she has ordered. i have not had any communication from my Queen, which likely means that i behaved in accordance to my Queen's wishes.

10:13 pm: Text from my wife. It is to advise me that a mutual friend wishes me to do a small job for her. i need to advise my Queen of this.

10:15 pm: i am angry at religion and the Church. We married as virgins, due to religious beliefs. It was an expensive decision – my wife has been an innocent party who has experienced great pain, only because i married without a great understanding of who i am sexually – i'd known of my submissive desires since childhood, but they were a larger part of me than i'd realised. Sex was a big disappointment to me. i found little pleasure, and could not obtain an erection. i then started to visualise Dom/sub thoughts to be able to perform.

MONDAY

8:14 am: Updated my Queen with my schedule for the day. i would be working today, but i begin a new job tomorrow. As such, i view today as a gift that i can devote to my wonderful Queen in the completion of her many tasks.

10:00 am: My Queen has called, very angry with me. She says that i am a pathetic creature because i revealed my favouritism between Mistress A and Mistress M. i must always serve all equally, and never disrupt their friendship. i have a leg fetish. Mistress A has very large breasts and Mistress M has small breasts but amazing legs. Obviously, i found Mistress M far more attractive. i suspect that Mistress A was a little jealous.

2:41 pm: My Queen has emailed me and ridiculed me for not providing her with details of the political constituency i am in. i feel very pathetic for i have completely forgotten about this. She needs this information to advise me whom i shall vote for in the general election.

4:09 pm: Text from a Mistress Large, telling me to keep Saturday free, and that we will not be alone. Not knowing adds to the fear, i guess. Since she has a fetish for seeing two men playing, i believe she will have a fuck buddy and she will make me watch them together. My Queen once told me that i must learn that all ladies are beautiful. She implied that i may not appreciate large ladies, and arranged that i serve Mistress Large.

4:11 pm: i do not usually serve Mistresses as frequently as this. Though i have always found it is like buses: you wait for one and then they all come together.

5:02 pm: i shall now go for my run in preparation for the marathon that my Queen ordered me to complete. i was initially shocked and afraid. Fortunately today is only be a five-mile run today.

6:33 pm: Supplying my Queen with my local results of the 2005 elections, so she has context to consider the situation.

8:19 pm: An email from Mistress A. She is very pleased with Saturday. However, she is annoyed that i sent her a text with text-speak. Because of this, she will take away my privileges: i shall not be permitted to sit and chat to her friends, but will serve them only. i shall miss these privileges greatly.

9:25 pm: i hate Facebook; it's so superficial. How long it takes due to the chats that i am not permitted to ignore.

9:29 pm: Just updated my Queen. i have not orgasmed in over ten days. It's getting harder each day.

10:45 pm: Served a Mistress online. A role-play communication. i had never done this before. She advised me that i must not tell anyone except my Queen.

11:00 pm: i have not heard from my Queen all night. In one sense it is good news, but the silence is painful. i remember when i would do something sloppy just to hear from her. But i have grown out of this, or rather, her training has improved my attitude and behaviour.

11:10 pm: Thinking of my Queen. When i told her that i needed to leave my wife, she warned me that i would be choosing a lonely, depressing experience. She also would not make any promises as to how long she will own me, and even indicated that she is getting bored of me, and may discard me after i separated. i was upset to hear this, but do not believe she will do the latter. i know my Queen may one day abandon me, but i desire and hope that she will allow me to dwell in her realm for the rest of my life. i suspect she wants to make sure i am leaving my wife for the right reasons.

TUESDAY

7:06 am: Last night i laid in bed and thought of my Queen. i did masturbate and i failed in that i did not refrain from orgasm. It was a self-imposed ban, for one day a Mistress or my Queen may choose to control this aspect of my life, and i need to become more disciplined.

7:08 am: My thoughts on my Queen have no sexual aspect. Here i must be careful, for i am forbidden to talk about my Queen – i can only discuss how she uses me. My Queen does not use me in a physical way. She sees me when it suits her. Sometimes, i dream of just lying with her, or looking at her beautiful face. i have not been permitted to look at her face for nearly two years now. i hate this. i live on the memory of our first meeting and her wonderful eyes. The last time i looked at her eyes, i felt an electrical surge run through my body. i experience this whenever she runs her hand through my hair or touches my knee.

7:13 am: My room is quite empty, as my Queen has stripped me of many of my possessions. i believe my Queen did this to teach me that real value is in people. i have always been in awe whenever i have heard my Queen speak to her friends on the phone. She makes everyone feel so special, and recognise their potential. She makes me realise how much power is in words. Sometimes i feel that i am her slave purely for this purpose – most of my tasks are promoting her friends' work.

7:30 am: Emailed my Queen, advising her that in my head i call her Beatrice, for Dante's love of Beatrice. i am not allowed to know her real name.

7:35 am: When i logged in to update my Queen, last night's online Mistress was also online. She reverted to the role play. So i guess it is ongoing?

8:30 am: Cycling to a special training at work. i am looking forward to meeting new people. But first, so many wonderful legs in stockings and heels of all types! One lady has high heels, the shortest skirt and seamed stockings. i got off my bike and walked behind her to admire the glorious sight without her knowing until she turned. Sheer joy and torture.

11:20 am: Finished a session with the head of HR. She is much older, and apparently comfortable with her sexuality. She wore sharply heeled, erotic shoes. Not work shoes. They were just amazing. Since i am rather cautious in nature, i shall wait to compliment her until i know it will only be taken the way it is meant. A sexy female is someone who is comfortable with her body and feels sexual. This is an important lesson our conventional society has lost.

2:34 pm: This is the first time i have worked for a large company. i opened my work's email box and nearly fell off my chair when i realised i have 734 emails there.

4:00 pm: Speaking with a colleague. i am considered to be fairly good-looking. That said within the BDSM culture, correspondence is always undertaken first. Looks, while important, are normally a secondary aspect. A good attitude and respect to the Dom/Dommes get you to the stage where consideration to your looks is made. Not so at work.

5:11 pm: Text from a Mistress telling me that i need to be put into chastity. Immensely excited.

7:41 pm: The training went well, i met many lovely people. i tried to replicate the attitude of my Queen by taking interest in each one. It is really an art.

7:45 pm: In the lady's Facebook account that i have to promote. It states it is her birthday today. i have so many messages to respond to. i hate Facebook.

7:56 pm: Two emails from my Queen, one reminding me that all people are worth more than i am, and one telling me which party i shall be voting for. i must research, to find out what to advise anyone who asks why i voted for them. She signed off 'Beatrice', which touched me deeply.

—⁓—

the fiery shopkeeper on an emotional roller coaster with her perfect long-distance boyfriend

35, FEMALE, BRIGHTON

SUNDAY

5:50 am: The text-message tone woke me up. Josh? Texting me to let me know he loves me, and can't wait to see me on Thursday? The alcohol-induced tiredness is too hard to shake. Can't get out of bed to check my phone. Sleep.

8:09 am: The 5 am text was not from him. It was from my friend Ben, wondering whether I know where to score drugs. Time to get up and go to work. On a Sunday! What a disgrace.

10:38 am: A man just walked into my shop. He wanted more than purchasing random stuff – he smiled the way men smile when they fancy me. When I was 20, my mum told me that it was okay to be fussy with guys. I was young, intelligent, pretty and I could afford to pick only the best. She also warned me that once beauty and youth wore off, I could no longer be fussy. I'd have to get what I could. At nearly 40, I finally understand what she means. I'm not married, I'm not a mother, my boyfriend is 6,000 miles away. I'm scared of looking back and having regrets.

12:05 pm: The shop is empty. After being single and wild for a decade, I found myself an *amazing* boyfriend… around the globe. In the beginning I thought a long-distance relationship would be exciting and different. After one year of expensive travels, I'm not so sure any more.

3:24 pm: He still hasn't texted. Not that I thought he would, after me behaving like a bitch yesterday. One of the many problems of a long-distance relationship: by the time he rang me, as soon as he got up in the morning, it was evening here and I'd just finished an 11-hour work shift. I also had PMS, and basically moaned non-stop for three hours.

7:00 pm: Went to the pub alone. Me! A pretty, young, funny, sociable, witty and interesting woman. Alone.

7:30 pm: Men are looking at me. I wish I could see the same desire in my boyfriend's eyes. He's more respectful and romantic than sexual – he'd never throw me on the bed and spank me.

11:00 pm: Yay! I danced! I drank! I kept my knickers on! Didn't puke in the street, though I peed in an alley. Success. I texted him all night, and got typical responses. I like it when he's a bit jealous. It shows passion. Right?

MONDAY

10:12 am: Ouch. Ouch. Ouch. My head is spinning. Sambucas. That's all I remember.

10:13 pm: Oh, I also remember that a gay man asked me politely whether he could touch my bum. Of course he could. I love being touched.

10:18 pm: This is, by the way, part of a pattern: My first days back from a visit are difficult to adjust to, it's when I miss him the most.

After the first week, I get into my routine: work really hard, plan my next two trips. My life is based around work and Josh trips. I get a bit wild when I do go out – I really do it heavily, going home and not knowing where I've been. See Josh. Repeat.

11:25 am: I haven't had sex for three weeks and two days. I am feeling horny. I'd love to think that when I see him next week, we'll spend the first day fucking like rabbits. But that's not how it works with him. He needs to be 'in the mood'. Why is it that every time I am in a relationship, I always feel I am the man?

12:00 pm: I've spent the week thinking that I should really end my long-distance relationship. So many problems.

3:30 pm: Thank god I have Pat, a little vibrator named after my boyfriend's middle name.

8:00 pm: Call from Josh, and I'm melting. So I do love him. This morning I wanted to leave him. This evening I want to propose to him.

9:54 pm: I think I am a freak. My friend says I am normal. But anyone who falls in and out of love 1,340 times a day is not normal. What do I need – a counsellor? A doctor? An exorcist? A personality transplant?

10:04 pm: I know what I need. I need a man who behaves like a man. Where I come from (the Mediterranean), men are really strong. They make decisions. I think a man should be a bit firm. Here they're weaker and more similar to women. My boyfriend is very laid-back. He will let me do whatever I want. He's respectful. I'm very feisty and fiery, and I want to meet someone who'll tell me, 'You can't do that!'

10:45 pm: And if I can't have that, I'll have a woman. If this doesn't work, this will be my last relationship with a man. If things don't work with him, they will not work with another man. Time to switch.

10:48 pm: To a woman like Victoria. She was only 19, fresh, beautiful, naughty and very keen. Usually that's a good combination for a great night. Except, I felt she was out of my league: her tits were far too perky, her lips were too sweet, her desire too intense. She said she had never been with a woman before. It didn't show. I now know what men feel when we are on top of them, riding them. I know how it feels to have the beautifully scented hair of a woman caressing your face. I know how empowered the men feel when they grab our hips. I know because two years ago, Victoria riding me happily throughout the night became the most divine thing I'd ever experienced.

TUESDAY

6:30 am: My alarm is a very unfunny joke. I can't possibly be so tired. I will not take a shower. I want to stink at work today.

12:02 pm: I feel guilty. Josh deserves more than me. He just called and told me he's planning a surprise vacation for us this weekend, because I 'worked so hard this month and deserve it.' I asked what the catch is, and he said: 'I love you! That's the only reason.'

12:04 pm: So, to recap, all the hours I've spent planning to leave him, he was planning a trip to make me happy. I. Am. Scum.

3:10 pm: Okay, lets liven it up a bit. I have no reason to be so bloody miserable all the time. I have everything a woman needs to be happy.

Well, perhaps not a fulfilling sex life, but I do have a man who adores me. And I'm not rich, but I can afford food every day, and Botox every six months. And the store's empty. So why the long face?

4:48 pm: Packing! For my surprise trip! What shall I bring? I don't even know where we're going. It will be like a honeymoon! This will be my chance to seduce him. I want to shock him. The problem is, I have fantasies in mind, but I get shy. He thinks I am a nice girl, but I am not a nice girl. I want to do something so that he can say, 'Ten years ago, she did _____ to me.'

4:49 pm: I know he likes porn, like any other man, but I wonder why he wanks over it, yet never wants to do the things he sees with me? Maybe I'm too innocent-behaving. Maybe I should do something outrageous. But how? Will anal sex do?

4:52 pm: He also doesn't believe I'm bisexual. When I point out nice-looking girls on the street, he looks at me like I'm just saying that to be cool. I don't think he understands that it's been going on since I was six years old.

7:31 pm: Talking to my mother on the phone. Josh and I have proven everyone wrong. We met when a friend randomly showed me a picture. I called my mother and said, 'I've met the man of my life.' It's difficult to explain – I just knew I'd marry him sooner or later. I decided that he'd be falling in love with me within the year. Later, we randomly met at a party (fate!). He did fall in love with me, and the amazing thing is that I only had to be myself. I am, after all, a really cool chick, if we put aside the OCD. (I colour-coordinate the soups in the cupboard. I bought a bathrobe to match my carpet. Little things.)

7:35 pm: He also puts aside my mood swings, anger issues, commitment phobia, sharp tongue and beer belly. I'm very passionate. I blame him, but I don't *blame* him.

9:44 pm: Next month we'll celebrate our first anniversary. All the things I saw in him in the photo were the things I discovered in him later. Travelling back and forth every month has worked so far, but we both know that the time to make a final decision is fast approaching. If we decide to be together, one of us has to move to another continent. And it's not gonna be me.

10:30 pm: Done packing! Clothes, shoes and accessories. But I'm dreading the jet lag, and the usual customs questions ('So you're dating a local? How's that work?' Answer: 'He won't move to my continent, and I won't move to his, so what's the point?' But how do you end a relationship with a man you still love and who loves you back?)

10:32 pm: Also dreading the first awkward moments in the airport, when I'm wondering whether Josh notices the new wrinkles.

11:15 pm: I can't wait to look into his amazingly tender blue eyes, smell his hair, laugh at his silly jokes, fall asleep to the sound of his voice. And I really – I mean, *really* – can't wait to finally get laid.

WEDNESDAY

9:54 am: Woke up wishing to be someone else. I fancy a change.

10:06 am: Considering the possibility of coming home from my trip as a single woman. How does this make me feel? Distraught, lonely and old. The idea of losing him makes want to cry until I drown.

2:39 pm: Just back from the beauty salon for a Hollywood wax. My pussy now looks like I have chicken bloody pox.

4:15 pm: Back from the hairdresser for a blow dry, and I look like an upside-down mop.

4:23 pm: Feel like a whale.

6:00 pm: Back home, where a card is waiting. From Josh, saying he can't wait to hold me. I've tried to snoop around and see if he has secret relationship, but he's just a nice man.

6:05 pm: Text from Josh, saying he's thinking of me. Trying to reply, but my fingers are frozen. It's the fourth week, and at this stage I drift away. I have no feelings, and can't say what I don't mean ('I love you').

9:13 pm: Whoever said that life begins at 40 should be shot. Gravity begins at 40. The changes in my vagina shocked the most. At 20 my vagina was my pride. So much so that I used to show it to anyone willing to take a look. With the same pride that mothers show photos of their children. Only I didn't have beautiful children, I had a beautiful vagina. Now? It's still neat, but when I wear tight jeans, my camel toe is bigger. I only show it during smear tests. I hope I die before I'm old.

11:45 pm: Bedtime positive affirmations:
1) I have an amazing, comfortable bed. Some people don't have a home.
2) I ate the most delicious pizza for dinner. Some people don't have any food.
3) My hair looks like a mop. Some people don't have hair.
4) Thank. God. For Pat.

THURDSAY

5:00 am: Awake for a taxi to the airport. I have no feelings whatsoever.

8:00 pm: Local time. The flight was so long, painful, and contaminated by many gloomy thoughts.

9:15 pm: Just sniffed by a sniffer dog! I thought I'd left a spliff in my bag, but it was only a banana.

11:00 pm: At Immigration. They saw that I've been here five times this year, and sent me to the Immigration Room. I didn't know the name of Josh's company, so it took an hour.

11:30 pm: Tense. Looking for Josh.

1:00 am: In Josh's bed! He's showering. We made love. I was expecting he would take me with fury. After all, full balls are full balls. But Josh took his time, seeming shy (or just detached?), and he was just so warm, his skin so soft. He's so sexy. The foreplay lasted longer than I wanted (though I constantly moan that it's not long enough), so I had to take matters into my own hands, quite literally. The result is a satisfactory orgasm and a smiley vagina.

FRIDAY

6:50 am: Waking up next to Josh makes me wonder what on Earth I was worried about. In his arms, I feel I belong.

8:00 am: Thinking about last night. Something was missing. And, surprise surprise, this time was not from me. Usually I am the one who's a bit distant in the beginning, a bit moody. It was a bit of a shock. Maybe this isn't going anywhere, and he's too gentlemanly to mention it? He's previously said that he finds it hard to cope with my mood swings and he's not sure if I love him.

9:00 am: Apparently time for the surprise short break! This morning! So happy!

2:00 pm: Oh my good Lord. Josh has reserved a room in the most wonderful chalet, up in the mountains, surrounded by snow. He has thought of everything, including upgrading our room to provide me with the most beautiful view. I am touched.

8:00 pm: We had sex. Great sex, rough sex, anal sex and now I can't even walk. My bum hole is in flames. Though I'm pretty sure I managed to shock him with my audacity, I'm not sure I will ever be able to poo again.

SATURDAY

9:00 am: Sigh. The weekend is briefer than we planned due to an approaching snow storm. We decided to leave before getting stuck, and besides, I need a pharmacy because my bum looks like a baboon. I'm gonna walk into a pharmacy and just tell the truth: 'Good morning, I recently had butt sex for the purpose of impressing my boyfriend, but I now suspect I need stitches, can you help?' Foreigners have anal sex too, right?

2:00 pm: Watching Josh drive. By sticking with Josh, am I choosing what I really want, or settling for the best possible choice?

3:00 pm: Josh just asked if he can read this diary. I said he could, but only after my death.

5:15 pm: In a way I believe that he's too nice for me, because deep down I know that I'm not a nice person. He's so nice that I hate him sometimes.

11:00 pm: Bedtime! Cuddle time! It's so cold tonight, perfect. I am most definitely continuing my relationship despite my constant doubts.

—∿—

8

SINGLES: UNCOMMITTED

the single gal who blames her love life on her height

31, FEMALE, LONDON

WEDNESDAY

1:06 pm: My flatmate just left. Finally! I can masturbate. Reading a couple of bondage stories on Literotica.com.

1:15 pm: I am currently single, and have been for a year. I only seem to meet guys who I either like as a person, *or* am attracted to. You'd expect a 31-year-old to have more interest in meeting a man, but I can't seem to bring myself to care. Ideally, I would just have a person in my bed. I miss physical contact.

2:00 pm: Can't seem to stop checking Jonathon's Facebook page several times a day, even though I think he is an idiot. It's just because he's the last person I slept with, five weeks ago – first sex I'd had in a year. So hot. Don't want to go out with him, but wish he would call.

2:03 pm: I think about our encounter in the bathroom all the time. I wouldn't normally agree to bathroom sex, but he was so insistent, and I was a bit drunk. It was like a scene from a porn film, all very dramatic and softly lit. And a bit difficult – small bathroom, two very tall people!

2:05 pm: I think if I can manage casual sex with someone I don't hate every couple of months, I might be able to stop obsessing about guys like Jonathon and focus on my career and not worry that I'm wasting all my good sex years alone. Need to avoid another year of unintentional celibacy.

3:44 pm: Just checked my profile on AdultFriendFinder.com, and both men I've been emailing want to meet me. One is mildly attractive, and his emails are readable. The other guy, an architect, writes less well, but is much better-looking. I've never done anything like this before, and I'm afraid of them wanting to meet up and me bottling.

5:06 pm: It's really easy to forget to go out and meet men when you have a Rabbit. And I'm having trouble having orgasms sometimes. I'm going to try and go a few days without using it.

11:08 pm: You want a bedtime secret? Here's one: when I was in university, I once gave a blow job to a taxi driver instead of paying him. I do stuff like this every couple of years, something that's really fucked up and out of character. Plus, I had the money! But he was cute, we were flirting, and I suggested it. My best friend knows.

THURSDAY

9:05 am: Very weird dream last night about the guy from the sex website, Aiden. He is very cute on the website, but in my dream he looked about 12 years old. I was not happy at being deceived.

12:10 pm: Email from Aiden asking me to describe exactly what I mean by wanting to meet a dominant man. Not sure what to reply. I'm not really experienced in all that sort of thing, just intrigued. I hope I don't disappoint him when we meet up. In truth, I've always wanted to try some hardcore bondage. That's why I joined the sex website.

12:11 pm: I think that's also why I've received responses such as: 'Let me rape your face.' Because I put that I like to be dominated. Still, face rape… that's a bit much.

12:15 pm: I should say here that I was not attractive when I was young. I am still about 15 in my head, that gangly tall girl nobody wants to go out with. I'm attractive now, or so I'm told. Things started to change around the age of 20. But I'm so utterly terrified of rejection or ridicule. I am passive, and wait for men to come to me, then pick one so busy talking about himself that he won't see that I'm not as great as he thought I was.

5:51 pm: Just got my period, so sex is the absolute last thing on my mind. I feel disgusting.

8:00 pm: I've just spent ages practising for a performance next week where I know I'll be seeing Jonathan, so I can impress him. And imagining what I'll say to him to make him think that I don't care (in a casual, non-combative way!), and to make him want to sleep with me again. It's tragic. I know other girls do this too.

10:00 pm: I thought many years ago that the man for me was Jimmy. I slept with him from the ages of 24 to 28. Then he found a real girlfriend. I was so in love with him, but as the years went by, I realised that he didn't really have any interest in me.

3:29 am: Tonight, I saw this guy, Phil, who plays with this band. He's been pursuing me for months, clearly interested, and a nice, funny, slightly weird guy. He would make a lovely boyfriend, but I try to imagine kissing him, and it just makes my skin crawl.

FRIDAY

12:35 pm: Just read an article about people who let nothing get them down, and I realised that I am the exact opposite of that. When I look at the past two years of my life, I feel disappointed. Because I really am an underachiever, and a total waste of potential.

1:00 pm: Spoke to my best friend Emily. I am worried we talk about being single too much. It makes me scared we're only friends because we're lonely. She says no, it's because we're so used to being single that our friendships become so strong. I like her answer better.

1:10 pm: We talked about Ollie, who I haven't thought about in months and months. We met at a gig – where else? – when he walked up to me and started talking to me. I very rarely choose my men, they just seem to choose me. It was all just so easy, suddenly, after years of being single, I was someone's girlfriend. I was crazy about him, mostly because he was crazy about me, and he was only crazy about me because he wanted someone to listen to him talk about himself, which I did, while grateful for the incredible sex. After we broke up I stalked Ollie for a year through Facebook and MySpace. It's horrific, the amount of hold technology has over you. You become a crazy person. But it was good that we'd stopped contact.

3:51 pm: I work alone all day as a freelancer. I am rejected all day and have no co-workers and I am desperately lonely because of that, and cling to human contact of any kind. I am running out of excuses as to why I'm so flaky and the real answer is that the work is so boring, it makes me question my own existence.

4:00 pm: Wedding tonight. I'm kind of ambivalent. I like Daniel – not mad keen on Laura, but I don't much care about their love.

7:09 pm: Waiting for people to arrive with Jack, whose loneliness is palpable, and Amy, who is as depressed as I am to be here. They've been my best friends for about ten years, and I am worried about both. Jack is really struggling with work and love, and Amy is Internet dating like a fiend because she's scared to be alone after a four-year relationship. I wish she'd calm down about it, because her fears are starting to make me feel scared too.

9:08 pm: Laura, the most annoying bride in the world – God I hate her – squeaking on and on about how perfect her relationship is. Wonder if she knows how bipolar Daniel is? Though, how could he keep it a secret?

9:10 am: I shouldn't be mean. She isn't a bad person. Just hideous company.

10:15 pm: Met a really cute guy outside having a cigarette. He was so into me when I told him I was a performer. But I just couldn't bring myself to get enthused, conversing was such an effort, I eventually stopped bothering.

10:40 pm: She just threw the bouquet. Me and Amy read each other's minds. I loudly said to Amy that I'd rather get fucked, flame first, through the eye with a lit candle than jump in to try and catch it. Got a weird look from a girl.

2:17 am: Don't know if this happens to anyone else, but if I'm mid-masturbation, the evil part of my brain takes over and throws really grotesque pictures into my head. Ruined an already upsetting evening.

SATURDAY

10:06 am: After last night's misery-wanking attempts, awoke from a sex dream about Idris Elba, the guy who plays Stringer Bell in *The Wire*. Managed to stay asleep long enough to enjoy it.

10:30 am: Thinking a lot about this guy Ivan, a very short, sexy black comedian. I am attracted to him, but have this problem with someone shorter than me. It makes me feel very unfeminine. Ideally, the man shouldn't be smaller than me. I have this image of myself made of pudding, and if the guy can fit his entire body inside my entire pudding body without any bits sticking out, then he's too small. I once had a connection with a guy called Lee – he was TINY. We both felt the connection, and we both felt the same way about the size issue. My friend Amelia says I am ridiculous. But she's 5'2".

12:30 pm: Lunch with my sister and husband, who told us they were separating a few months ago, but appear to be back together. Nobody talks about it.

9:02 pm: I am spending most of tonight worrying about not having a pension or savings, and thinking that if I end up one of those old ladies whose cat eats her face because she can't afford central heating, I am going to hoard sleeping pills and kill myself.

SUNDAY

10:44 am: Jonathan just emailed me about performing with him next week. It was an impersonal email, and I wrote an equally breezy impersonal one back. I want so much for him to take me home, and I worry that his army of fans will be there, and he won't choose me. I am SO TOO OLD for these thoughts. I will likely end up rejecting him first, even though I want the exact opposite. I am pathetic.

3:49 pm: I mostly helped my mum all day prepare for Passover. I am terrified that my mum will die. I'm 31, and I have been terrified of this for as long as I can remember. I think it's because she is the only person who has ever, or ever will, love me unconditionally. I hope that's not true, but it feels that way.

8:00 pm: My mum's friend Joanne was over for Passover. I've been seeing loads of her son because he plays guitar in my friend's band. He has a creepy squint but is basically an okay guy. I have this disgusting habit of imagining sex with people I find physically off-putting. I don't know why – maybe I still feel guilty about sex, the way my mother seemed to want me to. When sex would come on TV, she'd switch over and tell me, 'Nice girls don't do that!'

12:08 am: Watched Stringer Bell on *The Wire*. I'm not usually attracted to black men, but he's incredibly beautiful.

2:00 am: Jonathan emailed me back, and sent me into a spiral of self-doubt, but at least I'm old enough to realise that I'm probably reading things into it that aren't there. And if they are there, they don't really matter.

—⁓—

the sassy virgin student casing the library for 'the one'

20, FEMALE, WEST MIDLANDS

WEDNESDAY

11:47 am: At the library, have no idea why I've totally dressed up.

11:48 am: I do know why. Because there's a chance I'll bump into Irish, a guy that I kissed a few weeks back at my party, who never got in touch with me again. Had no problem keeping in touch with my friends, though. I don't regret him. He had an unbelievably cute Irish accent and very blue eyes. I'm Middle Eastern and live in London. A guy from Stoke or Dublin just seems so exotic.

2:14 pm: Cringe, cringe, cringe! Irish was sitting behind me, didn't acknowledge me. To be fair, nor did I. At least my hair looks pretty? It's so strange, all these random boys. My romantic sentiment leads me to believe there's a chance that 'The One' is here. Yeah, erm, definitely not in this library. Perception very distorted: 5/10s become 8/10s. Anyway, focus, very important, philosophy essay.

2:56 pm: Thinking about the random university hook-ups I've had (there have been eight the past three years, mostly very drunk). When I say 'hook-up', I really do just mean a kiss. None of them were actually worth it. Randomly kissing guys is just not very fun. I mean there is humour in it, but it is just that – random.

2:57 pm: Oh, and I suppose since we're on regret, another random hook-up: Indian, 19, south-east London, referred to me as a MILF.

2:58 pm: A proper introduction: I go to a prestigious but romantically dead university. You'll end up alone unless you're loose or markedly reduce your standards. And here I am: graduate this year, single and a virgin. I'm relying on the men in the future and not taking the present ones seriously. Sometimes I think boyfriends can thwart your growth.

3:01 pm: Such as Max. After six months, he got all my guards down, then told me he was falling in love. Then the following day he told me that we were too different, he loved his ex-girlfriend. We didn't speak for five months, ignored one another in seminars, and then I finally thought (while at a detox retreat doing a one-week juice fast) that I need to tell him how he made me feel (shit). So this past week we sort of hooked up, making out on his bed after he revealed his regret and intense want for me.

4:45 pm: God, I just have to tell you about one guy in the library. I sit here because I know he'll sit there. I've gathered that he and the beautiful girl he kisses are dating. He is just such a man – beard, amazing smile, like, he looks primitive in the very best way. I (and, okay, my gay best friend) just creepily stare at him the entire time.

9:05 pm: Can I just say, I AM ATTRACTIVE. I do not feel like a woman at this uni. We're watching the football match at the union, and we just suddenly got caught up in an UNDER-15 football tournament, and I think it was the first time I've been hit on at this university. They were 14-year-old boys and their line was literally, 'Blud it be haaaat in hee or wat ye, ye boi yeee haaat.'

9:08 pm: So yeah, GUYS: THE GIRLS ARE PROBABLY MUCH MORE WILLING TO REDUCE THEIR STANDARDS THAN YOU CARE TO BELIEVE.

THURSDAY

9:00 am: Phone call with my mother. My family is traditional Muslim. My mother wants to marry me off to a nice Muslim boy, but she is also a born-again feminist who thinks I should avoid boys until I've achieved my goals (Ivy League master's degree, travel, dream job, etc). I interpret her advice to fit my life, so when she's like, 'You should go out with a guy and hold hands,' I think, 'Mummy's given me the okay for third base.'

11:00 am: I have a routine: skinny latte and low-fat muffin, library. Routine, routine. I think it's healthy. I'm planning on waking up earlier in the mornings, as all my crazy decisions happen at night. Better to limit those hours. I'm not overweight but I am slightly chubby. This is not acceptable in my social circle. I'm always on a yo-yo diet. For a long time I thought I was single because of my weight until a guy fell for me in Asia in a big way. He was very hot in every way and we had a brief summer fling.

11:10 am: I've managed to persuade my best friend Storm from London to come study here with me. She's Jewish and understands the crazy traditional culture of my family. Looking around the library. No one good-looking. Our campus population was voted worst-looking in a nationwide survey. Caveman Fantasy Guy is not here yet. I am generally a nightmare to be sitting next to – I used to think I wasn't *that* person, with the music blasting through headphones, but yeah, I am.

11:11 am: France *has* to be better. It will be. I'm moving there next year. In nine months I'll be living in France, hopefully dating many eligible men and hopefully making love and being in love with some incredibly hot, very eligible man.

12:36 pm: A guy who looks like Skipper Johnston from *Sex in the City* thinks I'm interested. He keeps looking this way, I think, to see whether I'm looking his way, and I am. Vicious awkward library moment.

5:04 pm: Max and I are having quite an intense convo over Skype. He isn't happy about our situation.

5:10 pm: Now he wants me back. He fucked me over hardcore, though, so I'm not super-sympathetic. He reckons I'm giving him boundaries and he's open for business. I think it's time to clear things up!

5:09 pm: It does not help that we are talking in metaphors…

5:15 pm: Okay, so yeah, it's over. We're going to try and be friends (not that we were ever not just friends). He said I'm not a nice person. I can't even be bothered – it's boring. My sister, one of the most beautiful women you'll meet in real life, was in an on-and-off very messy Ross/Rachel relationship during her 20s and I suppose she's a warning: don't get trapped, if it's on/off, it's *off*.

FRIDAY

10:33 am: My sister just sent me this:

> *Emily Dickinson true, she is the archetypical spinster. But as a writer who (most likely) died a virgin, she's hardly without company – it's been rumoured that Lewis Carroll, Hans Christian Andersen, J.M. Barrie, Immanuel Kant, George Bernard Shaw, and William Butler Yeats all died virgins. Moreover, Emily didn't seem too upset about it, assuring a friend in a letter that she was not*

lonely: 'For my companions – the Hills, Sir, and the Sundown, and
a Dog, large as myself, that my Father bought me – They are better
than Beings.'

I don't know whether this is a good or terrible thing.

11:15 am: Library with Storm. Storm is also a virgin, so is Lily and so
is another of my closest friends. I suppose it is not that big a deal that
we're all 21 this year and not close to losing our virginity. I mean, the
vast majority of my friends would only sleep with someone in a
serious relationship. I suppose, though, I do find myself defending
my decision more, even if it's an internal battle. I just want to not
feel a sense of fatality towards the relationship.

11:23 am: I would, however, have sex with the following people:
Derren Brown and James Franco. I really don't need to be in a
relationship with those men. Also I think we are relatively secure and
happy, sex with the wrong guy just wouldn't be worth it for our self-
esteem. However, I do know that it's borderline creepy, like, okay, it's
sort of hot being a 20-year-old virgin but, I mean, what about 24? Is
that, 'So, what's her problem?'

11:37 am: You know the *Sex in the City* episode where the guy has a
closet relationship? He hides his girlfriend and, like, takes her to
these random restaurants. I think she was quite chubby. I feel a bit
like that jerk with Max. No! It's over.

11:59 am: I have a giant crush on a guy at this university. He doesn't
know me. He looks a lot like Derren Brown (my dream man, I've
always liked him because I felt like he was so interesting but I was 14
when it started), so his friend thought it would be funny after
hearing I have this whole Derren Brown obsession to have me send

him a weird FB message. I think I said, 'Hey, you look like Derren Brown, I really love him'. It wasn't clever or witty, just very embarrassing.

3:26 pm: Forced by Sarah and Storm to watch a depressing tween movie. My friends and I wish we were boys. We wouldn't be single because we have money. It's an awful thing to say, but I see my brother. He gets every girl he wants. I look at these girls and think, 'Are you stupid? Why would you stay with a guy who is so obviously riddled with issues?' I know some guys here get put off that I drive a nice car and have a nice watch.

8:30 pm: Sarah tells me Irish is outside pouring his heart out to his ex-girlfriend. I was just a ploy to get her jealous due to our similar ethnicity. I don't really care about that. I just wish I could know what it feels like to be in a real relationship, not obsessions and flings.

9:00 pm: Sarah is demonstrating her perfect BJ skills. It has to be said I have very few skills, and I sort of think I wish I had more practice. The honest truth is, I want to do everything and have my guards down with someone I truly love and trust. When the right guy comes, I'll try everything (but anal – no thanks) and I think I'll be very into it.

1:44 am: I hope Sarah is okay. She was going to message her 'must have no contact guy'. He treats her badly and just uses her. I, however, fell asleep at 12 am and never got back to her.

SATURDAY

9:45 am: Max just called, quite annoyed really, and asked, 'Who told you I was a bad boyfriend toward my ex?' Well, whether or not it's true, I would never reveal something a friend who told me something out of confidence. When I said as much, he screamed that I'm not a nice person for messing him around. SCREAMED. I'm not socialising with him. He is aggressive and thoughtless.

9:48 am: No one has the right to scream at anyone, I will not allow that. I want to say, 'Dude, I have priorities. I'm not going to bend my principles for you and your ego. THANKS.'

12:05 pm: Storm has left for London. Lily is off dating someone. I've been a very, very good girl, I'd like to think. I want to help change things in the Middle East. Only the opportunity cost means I have no romance in my life. It's so hard to find a nice guy, and Lily has.

12:20 pm: Library. I am sitting next to a guy I know. He is not attractive. But for some reason I am completely drawn to him. He is perhaps my biggest hidden crush. He is super calm and intelligent. There is mystery behind the long black hair, the beard, the skinny small frame and the thick-rimmed glasses. He doesn't believe in consumerism, so his dress sense is terrible. He's an anarchist. But I'm attracted. I don't understand how my mind works.

12:23 pm: Very sexy French guy just walked in. I know him through friends. He's amazing. Aahh, talk to meeeee. Alexandra would know what to do. You know you have some girls who just understand guys, just do the right thing and ooze their own unique confidence and sex appeal? That's Alexandra, one of my best friends. I'm only good on the phone, sort of cute and witty with my messages.

4:24 pm : Sarah and I are sitting next to each other and a MAGICAL thing has happened, a very pretty boy, with a jersey which has printed on his back 'ultra fag' has appeared. Not only is he pretty, the jersey proves he has a sense of humour. I think all women would like his eyes. They're big and hazel. He's deep in a book about Ireland (Sarah went to stalk). The truth is these magical men do appear in and out of our lives. By not actually having any real contact with them, our fantasies can be kept intact. I think he looks like an Asian prince.

4:33 pm: His Asian princess has arrived.

—⁓—

the gay journalist in a sexual drought following years of bounty

43, MALE, LONDON

WEDNESDAY

6:02 am: Awake. Wondering what to wear to the office today. Worried about my ever-expanding waistline. And worried I'll never have sex again.

6:05 am: I'm long-term single, and I'm not sure how that happened, as I was sexually busy in my 20s and 30s. I haven't had sex or a relationship in over two years. It's been so long since I had sex that it seems a ridiculous idea.

7:00 am: Letched after a guy running fast on the treadmill at the gym. I have a penchant for short, dark, bearded men, and for years lived in countries where I could hone that taste. I am equally taken with this guy's face and running style (effortless).

8:15 am: In the café having my morning cappuccino, fantasising about having a threesome with a couple of bearded guys at a table.

11:00 am: Sitting on a bench watching an amorous male pigeon. Each time a new female appears, he puffs up his chest and throws himself at her. And each time she flies away, rejecting him, he deflates his chest and pecks around until another female arrives. Then he starts the whole process again. I admire his determination.

12:57 pm: Just had my printer fixed by a sexy IT bod. Which sounds like an oxymoron. It's not.

4:15 pm: Email from my ex. We were together for 16 months. It was glorious at first – the joy of discovery, feeling attractive again and feeling 'normal' for actually having a partner – but we were too different to make a go of it. Also, I worked; he spent. We remain good mates.

6:13 pm: Dinner with my friend Andrea, who thinks she is splitting from her boyfriend after 18 years. Dinner is so-so, company is nice. She thinks that I just need some time to be my own person, after being in relationships pretty much constantly since I was 17. But look where it got me! Feel fat and bloated.

10:58 pm: Flatmate is, I think, having a Gaydar shag in his room: front door was locked, but the TV is on and there are signs of life (wallet, bag, etc).

10:59 pm: Yes, Gaydar shag. His laptop is not in its usual place, which makes me think they are probably having a porn fest. Rather him than me! I'm off pornography now. It started to feel a bit wrong and exploitative, and not in keeping with my newfound spiritual approach to life: Buddhist-with-a-twist. (The twist: I wear leather and I booze.)

11:15 pm: This said, can my new approach to life actually get me where I see myself? In a lovely home with someone I consider to be my soulmate?

THURSDAY

5:54 am: Up, fretting about how much I have to do, and worrying that I will indeed never have another sexual relationship because I'm so hung up on my body. Sometimes it takes up almost all my time trying not to think about it.

6:35 am: Commute. I feel like the Invisible Man, like no one ever looks at me and thinks, 'Oh, he's cute.' I'm on Gaydar and Manhunt, but never get so much as a glance. I'm not saying that in a 'poor me' way – I don't suffer from I'm Hideous-Looking Syndrome (thank God, where would I find the time!), but just stating a fact. I've had a couple of coffees with guys I didn't click with, and that's it.

10:56 am: Two coffees but seriously flagging at work. Wondering what kind of wardrobe to buy: my temporary one is about to collapse. I know how it feels.

10:57 am: I seem to be dwelling on how unattractive I am. I wonder if thinking that men don't fancy me is a self-fulfilling prophesy?

11:39 am: Taking a break on the street. I can hear people talking to their other halves on mobile phones. I wonder where all these people in relationships all meet each other? Most of my mates seem to have met people through work.

2:45 pm: Just had an alarming email from my flatmate saying he needs to get something off his chest re: house thing. Oh dear.

4:23 pm: Just interviewed a menswear designer. Need new clothes. I've got some nice pieces, but have been out of the spending circuit for a while and feel like loads of my clothes are dated. Do people even wear my beloved silver Converse any more?

8:16 pm: Lovely dinner with Abby, an ex-colleague who I haven't seen for far too long. Talked about work and love. And she is going to give me her wardrobe, which is marvellous and will save me both money and commitment issues. Hopefully I won't have to wait too long, because my temporary tent thing is going to collapse any second now.

10:12 pm: Almost considered popping into a gay bar on the way home. Didn't do it. Now sitting on the sofa watching bad TV. I'm generally okay with my single status, though sometimes I would really like to come home to someone giving me a cuddle. I also worry sometimes that I will never have sex again, much less hear someone tell me they love me.

12:12 am: What my flatmate wanted to get off his chest: that I need to get myself some Viagra, and get on with it. It was nice to speak frankly about my total lack of sex life with another man.

12:24 am: Thinking about the days when sex wasn't such a weighted and complicated gay issue. When I was younger I used to be versatile when it came to fucking. I am now a total bottom due to the fact that I can't maintain a hard-on when topping, especially when wearing a condom. Wish I'd done more topping while I could. Never been interested in the extremes of gay sex like fisting, CP* or watersports (though I did experiment with golden showers with one boyfriend, and it was okay). I might have liked to have had a bit more group sex.

---

* Corporal punishment.

FRIDAY

4:30 am: Awake, as per, but actually with a hard-on, which is increasingly rare. I wank a couple of times a week, more to keep my hand in than out of any pressing need. I read that as you get older you need to ejaculate regularly for health reasons.

7:00 am: Listened to Radio 4, got up and did a sit, then went out for a run round the common. My preoccupation with my belly continues. It's a full-time job. As usual had to force myself to do it, and then loved it. Though I am currently suffering from a foot injury, so a lot of my time is spent fretting about the roll of gathering midriff flab. Fat family genes and middle age obviously don't help.

2:14 pm: In East London. I see most males as 'yes I would' or 'no I wouldn't' before I actually really see them. The street is full of skinny jeans and young males with odd moustaches. Making me feel old.

4:44 pm: Just back. Wrapped sister's birthday present, did a face-pack and put up a mirror.

6:43 pm: Bantering with someone on Thingbox.com about how miserable he is following a break-up. Weird how you can get into intimate conversations with people you've never met and then never speak to them again.

6:55 pm: Curtain-twiching* on Gaydar. No tracks. And no one I like the look of.

7:15 pm: Going to cut my hair, while thinking about all the things I'll tell Jordi at our next talk. We talk two times a year. He's

---

* Looking at user profiles invisibly.

probably the love of my life. We lived together in a lovely flat for four years, 15 years ago.

8:20 pm: Met my sister Jackie, and her weird, fat friends, one of whom refused to walk from Embankment to Convent Garden. Jackie is one of my best mates, and probably my spiritual soulmate. (This is different from my mum, who's probably the non-sexual love of my life. Spot the gay cliché!) Funny how we've all turned out so differently. I wonder what we would make of each other if we met randomly.

9:00 pm: Eating too much curry, talking about my dad. He was a serial philanderer, I was privy to his affairs from an early age, courtesy of my mum. This has shaped how I feel about relationships: the inevitability that one or both parties will stray. Compounded by the fact that my first great love was unfaithful. And thus why I go into a massively insecure mode at the beginning of a relationship.

9:02 pm: Yes, I'm talking as someone who has played around in relationships.

10:15 pm: Lovely evening back in north London. We drank too much. My consumption is creeping up again. And of course there's the summer-holiday beer belly beach body to think about.

11:00 pm: Jackie pointed out some new veins on my leg. My first varicose veins. Another thing to fret about.

11:30 pm: Tube. Letching first at a cute Eastern European-looking guy on the train who has the biggest bulge I've seen in a long time; now at another cutie with a dark goatee, who I think might have given me the eye. As with pigeons, so with humans.

—◠◠—

the porn-loving, long-time bachelor who's just fine alone, thank you

49, MALE, LONDON

FRIDAY

8:39 am: On the Tube. Usual assortment of semi-attractive women, including one lovely blonde. Unfortunately she's flat-chested, and worse, clearly a bit dim: she's clinging to the high handrail, when she could hold onto the pole with much less risk of a dislocated shoulder.

9:45 am: Hot office topic: which trainees were disciplined for getting jiggy after too much sauce at a department drink-up earlier this week? I have often got drunk on the premises, but never have come close to indulging in shenanigans. Shame.

9:48 am: One exception: I remember leaving a 2002 do where I unsuccessfully tried to snog a buxom German blonde, much to the amusement of several onlookers.

1:54 pm: Bumped into Alana in a restaurant, a happily married mother who I fancied like crazy when I first met her. We have a mildly flirtatious relationship. She was asking for advice on how to do a performance report on a co-worker. I told her to try writing, 'She should be more like Alana.' How can I be this smooth and still single?

3:35 pm: Just had my annual job performance review, at which I gained an 'outstanding' rating for my administration work. Good thing private lives do not have the same sort of review. I'd be 'poor' or 'needs improvement.' Haven't been in a relationship in years, not sure whether I miss it. Do, however, miss the sex.

6:53 pm: A friend just asked me how I am. I suspect my friends desperately want me to say, 'I'm in a new relationship!' Are they disappointed that I am not in one? People tell me I am so nice I should be in one. Being nice seems like a good reason *not* to be in one. The person I am in a relationship is not favourable.

6:57 pm: This is how I would like to answer: 'Dear Friend, in the future, I will be exactly where I am now: not in a relationship. I hope to have at least some sex with someone. Ten years from now, I hope to have had sex with lots of people to make up for lost time. But I do NOT see myself in a relationship. Ever.'

7:31 pm: Why did I join that dating website, Match Affinity? Am now overrun with emails by supposedly compatible women, none of whom sound compatible.

7:34 pm: I am not in a relationship because I am pretty sure I am rubbish at them. All mine have had dysfunction, and I become too focused, to the detriment of my friendships. I also try too hard to impress the person. However, it has been so long that I can no longer be 100 per cent sure.

9:07 pm: Back from a walk. Wonder if it is the effect of that dating website, but I seem to notice more and more attractive women of my age group. I would describe myself as Black British, and I have never fancied anyone from my own ethnic group. Perhaps something to do with not wanting to end up with someone who might remind me of my mother. As I have put on weight, I have developed more of a taste for plumper women. Have to face the fact that a size-10 woman with a 300-pound boyfriend just looks freakish.

SATURDAY

10:45 am: The biggest turn-off in porn is a woman with legs slimmer than my arms. (Am I kidding myself to think that wanking over women who do not conform to models' shapes is somehow less pathetic?) A woman on a porn website automatically becomes a figure of fantasy, even if her body shape is one that most women on the street have.

10:48 am: My taste in porn is geared toward bigger women. 'Rubenesque' is a key word. Beth Ditto would be the largest woman I find attractive. Curvaceous, large breasts, slim waist, broad hips. Marilyn Monroe. Always remember that Marilyn was a size 16.

1:27 pm: Amazing how having my head shaved takes years off my look, so there is no grey, and no thinness of covering. I have not noticed a different response. Though when I grew a beard, there was a marked and positive response from female colleagues, who said it made me more 'dangerous', less cuddly, more sexy. Or so they said. Nobody actually left their husband as a result.

4:03 pm: No British man would think of Saturday as a day to mull over relationships. So my Saturday is all about the horses and the football.

5:45 pm: Feeling curiously disconnected from the afternoon's horse racing, which is rare. Wondering what else I might be doing, and whether a relationship would make any difference. We were together for four years, including a hiatus. We split in 1987. She, in particular, didn't put me off relationships.

6:17 pm: A roast loin of pork with lentils and bacon, and a nice glass of red wine. Food is my form of pampering myself, rather as some would eat chocolate or take a long bath.

9:26 pm: If I spent as much time having sex on the weekend as I do wanking, I would not be able to walk. I tend to masturbate in the mornings after rising, with occasional other sessions as the mood dictates. Masturbation is like all other sex: dull if routine. And I do have a bit of a routine.

SUNDAY

9:30 am: Watching my fair share of porn makes me want to try a few things: using a vibrator on a lover during anal sex, for a double penetration experience; experimenting with food and drink, like licking champagne; spanking; and I would not dismiss anal sex out of hand, giving or receiving. I think porn's made me more open to more things.

9:32 am: The above-mentioned dream about anal sex and a vibrator: the woman in my dream is a tall, leggy Eastern European blonde with whom I worked. She was implausibly beautiful, but like many Eastern European women, hopelessly self-obsessed and princess-like. I asked her out, she said yes, then stood me up. I don't set the score by dreams, but I do wonder if this one means something.

9:42 am: I worry that my use of pornography has left me incapable of 'proper' sex. I do realise that sex for a camera is very different than how most people have sex. I can't ask anyone because, well frankly, what are they going to do about it? It's not as if they can actually help.

10:55 am: Planned to hit the shops in the West End after a gym visit, but discovered as I arrived at the gym that I had forgotten my membership card. No gym visits = no weight loss = zero physical attraction = no sex/relationship = potential low self-esteem.

11:07 am: A gorgeous, sunny day, which brings out gorgeous women by the truckload. Am I destined for another summer of salivating?

6:42 pm: Wondering whether having one's team win is better than good sex, and a loss worse than bad sex. Whatever joy winning brings, I have never had sex bad enough to compare with Arsenal losing.

8:57 pm: I have a pile of ironing to do, Bach organ music and a cup of coffee. Would this be any more bearable if I had someone to talk to and occasionally cuddle? Boring tasks are boring tasks, and drawing someone else into them is just that.

MONDAY

7:30 am: Awake in my empty bed. Being single is comfortable enough to make me wonder why anyone would crave a relationship, other than to halve the rent and get ready access to sex. I cannot see how it is worth possibly hurting another person in order to find out.

7:32 am: I suppose it is just as likely that I could make someone incredibly happy. This is the one area of my life where I am a total pessimist.

8:49 am: Tube. Buxom beauty three feet away. She reminds me of Bea, a co-worker I once subbed for, with a chunky figure and delicate features. I'm wondering what it would be like to kiss her. She is a prime example of my taste in women, being bright, bubbly, curvaceous and very pretty. Bea was 20 years younger than me, but her parents had a similar age gap, so I asked her out. She very sweetly turned me down.

9:30 am: Feasting my eyes at work. I am proud of myself for taking a new job which has entailed making new friends, the majority of them extremely attractive women. If I really wanted a relationship, I could probably find someone at work.

11:30 am: Trying to reset the 'vibrate' settings on my phone, and wondering if anyone has ever stuck a mobile phone down the front of their pants, then got someone to ring them.

3:08 pm: Today's word of the day on my computer is 'scapegrace', which means 'a reckless scoundrel'. I would like to be a sexual scapegrace, if only for a few days, in the sexual sense. I'm sure this is exactly what the Word of the Day creators had in mind.

3:42 pm: A friend just emailed asking if anyone is interested in taking on a woman who is 'playful, inquisitive and likes to be handled'. Except I misread 'woman'. It was 'kitten'.

9:40 pm: Apparently my dating website profile does not say enough about me, and has been rejected by the site. Maybe there isn't much to say. Social networking is just another way to get rejected, only by so many more people.

9:58 pm: I have taken myself off the dating website. 'If it really is only the sex I miss, why bother fooling myself or anyone else? I should just bite the bullet and join a straightforward sex site.'

10:10 pm: Masturbated, to a repeat fantasy of making love very slowly, to *Discreet Music* by Brian Eno (no idea why), to my boss in a St Katherine's Dock or West End flat. It is odd to me that these fantasies all seem to derive from other, non-sexual, 'lifestyle' fantasies, like seeing an apartment on an estate agent's website and wondering what it would be like to live there.

TUESDAY

9:36 am: At work, researching sexual encounter websites. Thinking of the correct phrase to put into Google. Might be a sign that this is really not my style. And neither are soppy dating websites. Sort of between a cock and a hard place.

9:46 am: It's Connie's birthday tomorrow. She is physically perfect: statuesque, curvaceous with delicate features and a lovely soft voice, and also a very sweet, kind person. Can't shake the idea that she sort of fancies me. Like Alana, she has a flirtatious twinkle in her. Still, no point in being fancied by a married woman with two kids. In my experience, mothers shy away from affairs for fear of losing their children, so I do not live in hope.

1:08 pm: Nooooooooooooooooo. I just found out that my third-floor belle, Lottie, is on gardening leave, pending her move to another firm; I'd already heard that my second floor fancy is about to decamp abroad. I loved the twinkle in Lottie when she said hello. Am beginning to take this eye-candy exodus personally.

2:51 pm: Did some research and discovered that contact mags, which carry personal ads from people wanting to meet up purely for sex, have definitely migrated online. Seems much more honest than faffing around with dating websites.

—⁓—

the adorable consultant with an array of paramours, none of them mr right

33, FEMALE, SURREY

WEDNESDAY

8:00 am: I have date tonight! With Mr Match. I re-joined Match.com yesterday. Last time I joined, I met my now-ex on holiday a week later. So yesterday rejoining was easy because my profile was there, and all I had to do was add new photos.

1:00 pm: So last night I was browsing profiles of men and had nearly given up hope of finding anyone I was remotely interested in, when one profile jumped out at me. Mr Match: his good looks, blue sparkly eyes and big smile. His profile made me laugh (literally out loud!) and mentioned common interests and values. So after a bold first-move email on my part, we started chatting on IM, and before I knew it we were arranging for a drink. Am excited, and a bit nervous too.

3:00 pm: Text from Mr Match. Suddenly feels real now. My first date since breaking up with The Ex three months ago. And I haven't even decided what to wear.

5:00 pm: Trying to stay calm and not over-think date tonight with Mr Match. Part of me is *really* excited after such great chat on IM, and every time I look at his photo my stomach does flips. It feels like he is smiling right at me! But then other part of me thinks that something will go wrong. Can't be this easy.

6:30 pm: Why are there so many short-arse men on Match.com? A man has to be taller than me. Preferably over 6', but will put up with 5'9". Just.

11:48 pm: Just left the date! We chatted easily, but not the sparks I was hoping might fly. Though experience with The Ex indicates that instant fireworks can be bad in the long run. I think this might be a slow burn.

12:30 am: Back from my date. Felt really horny when I got into bed and masturbated while fantasising about what might happen on a future date.

THURSDAY

9:30 am: Even if my mind was not so sure about last night, my body was more sure.

11:23 am: Is it a bad idea to get back with an ex? Thinking about a guy I dated briefly early last year, who I ended up in bed with a couple of weeks ago. We get on really well, and are going on holiday together with a group in a few months. He slept the entire night with his arms wrapped around me, and it felt very intimate.

2:00 pm: Just had a massage, which was fantastic. All men should learn massage and sensitive touch. If a man I fancied touched me like that and then carried on…

4:30 pm: I fancy one of my colleagues, Michael, like mad, and he just asked if I wanted to join him and others for a drink after work. Yes yes and yes.

6:00 pm: Finishing work, and have arranged second date with Mr Match. We will go out near my place. Now pondering what the specific plans should be, and whether I will make any suggestion about him staying over at my place. Better tidy up just in case.

9:00 pm: At the pub with Michael, and he is being very flirty and tactile.

12:05 am: Just leaving the pub. When I started to leave, Michael 'confiscated' my train ticket. Unfortunately this man is married. So, much as it disappointed me to do so, I asked for my season ticket back and said goodnight with a peck on the cheek.

12:22 am: On the train. Feeling quite horny and flustered, and am having wicked thoughts of getting off and trying to get myself an invite back to his hotel. Why couldn't I feel like this about Mr Match, who is really keen on me and *single*?

1:05 am: Second night in a row home past midnight! What is it about something you can't have just making you want it more? Forbidden fruit. Am feeling really horny. I will just have to satisfy my horny feelings myself before I go to sleep.

FRIDAY

11:37 am: Just a lie-in and then working from home today. Question of the day: Should I be more proactive about my love life, or leave it to fate?

6:00 pm: Dinner with my parents, who are supportive of my status of being single. It does, however, make me question *why* I am single. Seventy or 80 per cent of my friends are in couples. This said, I am not sure there will ever be a single love of my life. I have so many loves in my life. Life is all about variety. Monogamy can work within some relationships, though I'd prefer my partner to be honest about what makes him or her happy. (And yes, I have had several close and sexual friendships with women, but no one who I have actually called my 'girlfriend'. I am open to the idea.)

10:00 pm: Just had a quick look on Match.com hoping that Mr Match might be online. He is probably out, rather than sitting in watching TV with his parents like I am.

12:42 am: Well Mr Match might not be online, but Mr Rugger Bugger is! He's a rather dashing rugby-playing older man. He has a lot going for him, so I'll forgive that he's the same height as me.

1:15 am: His direct questions about sex make it quite obvious what his motivation is. He is nowhere near as funny or lively a chat as Mr Match.

SATURDAY

6:39 pm: I've begun a rather spontaneous evening with Mr Rugger Bugger. We're at a pub for a few drinks near his house. By the standard of the pub, he is certainly not trying to overly impress me.

7:00 pm: Mr Rugger is buying me strong drinks, claiming that I 'need to catch up', as he's already had quite a few. I tell him that if I drink them, I will not be driving home. He says that's fine, he has spare rooms.

7:45 pm: In the toilet. We were just kissing, with him being very direct and forward. I think we both have a good idea that we'll end up in bed together.

10:30 pm: At Rugger's! He's downstairs. When we got back to his place, almost as soon as we walked in the door, his hands were under my shirt, undoing my jeans, down my jeans. He suggested that we go upstairs, and I didn't need asking twice.

12:00 am: We both took our clothes off and immediately were on the bed together. It was slightly strange experience in that, yes, I was physically enjoying it, but I had very little emotional connection or desire to jump him. I was just enjoying what he was doing to me. He was good with his hands and soon made me orgasm.

SUNDAY

9:23 am: This morning we picked up where we left off, this time with him fucking me with a bunny vibrator. We didn't have sex, but we did have lots of fun. Three orgasms for me!

9:45 am: Four. While Rugger was in the shower and taking ages, I helped myself to number four.

10:30 am: He just offered to take me out for breakfast, so we're off in his Porsche, which is very smart! Breakfast conversation is fine but not enthralling, all a little bit awkward somehow.

1:20 pm: I think he's hoping for round three, but I really can't be bothered. I just left, and feel very ambivalent, knowing that he's not someone I want anything long term with, or someone I feel likely to befriend. Unlikely I will see him again.

1:25 pm: I should add that this morning Rugger started asking quite a lot of questions about whether I get tested for STDs, when was the last time, how often, etc. This seemed an odd line of questioning since we hadn't had sex, and that I'd clearly said that if we did at any point, it would be with a condom. I wonder if he hopes that by telling me he gets tested regularly, I'll have unprotected sex with him?

9:00 pm: A bit worried that might have either bit of thrush or cystitis. Grrr. Feels funny when I pee. Better buy some cranberry juice.

9:50 pm: The more I think about it, the more I think I will not see Mr Rugger Bugger again. Although it was fun and there was physical attraction, I think all he is after is sex. Fine, he didn't make any secret of this, and I still felt in control of the situation. The conversation was nearly entirely around sex.

10:15 pm: Really nice text from Mr Match saying he is looking forward to our date. He has looked up trains and when they run back, so I'm glad he is not assuming that he is staying over.

MONDAY

11:50 am: Dinner booked with Mr Match for tomorrow night at 8 pm, at a really nice Thai restaurant, followed by a few drinks at pub with outdoor courtyard and live DJ. Feeling excited about it now. I have a 6 pm phone meeting with America, so I'll have to rush home!

2:10 pm: I was a little worried last night when there was obviously blood in my pee, as could be seen on toilet roll. But fortunately seems better today and although feels a bit funny, definitely better. The irony – Mr Rugger Bugger seemed obsessed that I'd been tested for STDs, and then caused me problems from basic hygiene.

2:15 pm: Some reading about cystitis, followed by thinking about it, leads me to reckon that the cause was him not being careful about where he was putting his fingers: they had been in my arse, and then went in my pussy. So it was probably that rather than the vibrator, which had been washed.

7:50 pm: In addition to the cystitis issues – which seem better now, phew! – I also now have what I think is a cold sore. Damn him.

8:30 pm: New guy at work is quite cute – and remembered me from a video about the company that I appeared in. Hmmm, potential? Maybe. Exceptions to mixing business and pleasure could be made for the right single person. Yet to find that out.

—⚬—

the post-divorce counsellor in search of less therapy and more sex

68, FEMALE, LONDON

WEDNESDAY

7:00 pm: Home. I'm not feeling sexual much at the moment. I can't remember the last time I masturbated. A few weeks ago? I need to be in the house on my own, as I need to make noise. Hearing myself making noise and saying dirty phrases always makes the feelings more intense. Fantasies, my own or borrowed, are very helpful too. The mind is the most erotic organ!

7:04 pm: I need to find that sexual energy again, as it lifts my mood and energy levels. Sex doesn't seem so important at the moment. The less I have, the less I want! I went for eight or nine years without it in the last years of my marriage, which ended four years ago. Sometimes being single seems a blessed relief and a kind of freedom.

9:34 pm: I'm tired now but feeling happier than last night when I was working far too late. In a few months, I'm stopping my work as a counsellor for retirement, and I'm dealing with both my patients' anxieties and my own. What a relief to stop, though! Enough for today. Goodnight.

THURSDAY

9:03 am: An overnight email from Nic. Soon after my marriage ended, we had a passionate affair which blew my mind. We were both making up for lost time and had great sexual chemistry, and a great mental rapport. Eighteen months ago he moved far away, and although we saw each other every six months, it wasn't enough for either of us. I needed to get on with finding someone here. He has a girlfriend now. It was a bit complicated when I visited last year, as none of his friends liked her. They have a relationship with plenty of space – i.e., they don't live together. So that is that.

11:13 am: I've just been looking on my Internet dating site, which I've used for some months with very little success, and found someone who looks very interesting and doesn't live too far way. I've sent an email, and fingers crossed he'll respond. This is the first time I've felt so optimistic about someone. He had a voice recording which sounded warm and interesting. I'm trying not to look for a 'Nic Replacement', but he was such a great lover. The next person I find has *a lot* to live up to. I did a lot of things with Nic: anal, fellatio, various permutations and positions, all very enjoyable. He liked to spank me, and we talked about how deeply he was penetrating me and filling me up. Also he would mock tie me up at times. I'm not going to settle for someone who doesn't interest and excite me.

2:56 pm: Looked in the mirror, and looked a bit haggard. How much older I feel because of minor health concerns and lack of any potential partners. So this is what getting old feels like! I realise that it is good to keep looking, and focus on what I do have. (Cliché, but true.)

4:00 pm: Online again. It is odd, like shopping for men. I'm realising that I need to stop searching for men so similar to me. My husband was very similar to me (upper middle-class, same ethnicity). He was attractive partly because he seemed like good breeding stock. I can't believe I'm writing this. He was bright and good-looking. No big challenges except in his sexual difficulties. He was younger and a virgin, whereas I had had a couple of year-long relationships and adventures/disasters. I recently expanded my search categories, and that has resulted in some interest.

4:15 pm: Hmmm. One man is perhaps too old at 79. Another seems interesting, but I'm already emailing and talking on the phone to a third man who seems quite interested. I sent him a long email on Sunday. At first I felt quite hopeful and had a few fantasies about what it might be like to get some sexual contact with him. But he doesn't say much about his interests or respond to what I've told him. I realise that I need to feel interested in him as a person to feel sexual, and that isn't happening.

5:00 pm: Chatting to my child's partner, who is lovely, and keeps me updated on my child. It reminds me that I do miss having a special person to care about and share thoughts and feelings.

5:50 pm: Had a brief nap and felt quite sexy. Nice after feeling so tired and dull for a weeks. Since Nic left, I've been single, I've kept myself busy with family concerns, work and friends. Counselling is a rather female-dominated world, and I look forward to having more attention for searching for a companion.

9:05 pm: Meal out with neighbours. One gay friend who is just 70 and couples. Lots of chat about dentistry, holidays and our children's generation and how selfish they are. I drank more than usual and that carried me through.

FRIDAY

8:00 am: Restless night, because a new medication is still affecting me.

12:14 pm: Just invited a friend and husband round for tea next week. I dread inviting them round because they do everything so properly – I feel a bit of a shambles in comparison – and they are very coupley, doing everything together now that they are retired. They are also opinionated. Since my husband left, I have learnt to stand up for my own views. I mustn't become a recluse because I'm not in a couple.

2:02 pm: My therapist just asked me about my sexual fantasies! I told her they will remain a secret because part of their sexual charge *is* secrecy. I hold them to myself to keep them mine: they have been about sex with a fantasy animal or beast, and about sex with a stranger ripping off my clothes. Nic used to call himself 'the beast', which pleased me.

5:42 pm: Feeling flat and tired. My day went a bit haywire because my car exhaust broke. Spending an hour getting it fixed threw out my trip to the rubbish tip. I also fitted in an extra session with a patient.

7:00 pm: Dashed through busy traffic to see my child and my child's family. I mucked in and helped a bit, cooking some food.

8:30 pm: Grandkids got tearful at bedtime. Exhausting! Not sure how much help I was.

11:00 pm: Responding to Nic's email. I still think about him very fondly. I had a sense of my mind expanding when with him – I guess you could say he's the love of my life. The sex was wonderful and memorable. I remember a passage by Chimamanda Adichie where a character talks of her lover taking her to 'another country'. I experienced that many times with Nic. Something transporting and blissful. There's no doubt that I was in love with him. Time to fall into bed.

—⁓—

the religious teacher aspiring to break the 'touch' barrier with his crush

23, MALE, BERKSHIRE

FRIDAY

10:00 am: Woke up really late and am now rushing to get to work. Today is the last day of a student holiday week. Excited to see Suzy, and looking forward to going out with her and Ella later.

10:01 am: I usually use holidays to get Suzy out of my head a bit. It is clear that I have failed miserably. I started working at my current school three years ago and met Suzy, and we slowly started to go out socially; when Ella arrived this year, we started to go out more. I was in another relationship until nine months ago. Still feel regret for the way that ended, and know I need to say sorry for that.

12:15 pm: Arrived at school and Suzy is running late. More annoyed about this than I should be.

3:00 pm: Suzy has arrived and we've had a long chat about bits and bobs. I always want to reach out and touch her. Never do.

6:12 pm: Didn't get half my work done, and now at Ella's. I'm a recovering fussy eater, and can now add fajitas to my list of foods that I eat.

9:30 pm: Really great conversation over dinner and wine. I always hope that wine will loosen up the situation so that I can say what I *feel*, not what I *think*. When there's logic involved, there has to be justification and thought process. But when I just say what I feel, there's no comeback, really.

11:30 pm: Just got in from pub near Ella's, and have had fun trying to sort bed out with Suzy and Ella. Bit of a wrestling match to get covers out of cases. Very sad to realise that this is probably the first time that I have touched a girl in nine months. It's a very stark thing to realise, and makes me want to change.

11:35 pm: What if I'm like this forever? Know that I'm a good(ish) person and I would really like to share that with someone, but I'm never able to get over those first few steps to show these good things off.

SATURDAY

8:09 am: Am quite hung-over, and woke up stupidly early.

8:30 am: Having a cup of tea with Ella while she's in her dressing gown. Doesn't do anything for me; she's like a big sister. Thinking about Suzy upstairs, on the other hand…

8:46 am: Suzy just woke up and came down in her pyjamas. She is at the other end of the sofa and all I can see is her bum. Really hard to concentrate.

10:30 am: Suzy just drove me to the station. We chatted about everything and nothing, and I'm slowly realising that we will never be a couple. I can see that what we have isn't necessarily romantic or fireworks, but just good solid conversation. It's not ideal, but it's okay.

10:45 am: On the train. Realising that I'm just too nice. This sounds lame. Suzy needs someone who is going to really argue with her. I've never quite worked out social boundaries when playful banter is called for.

12:30 pm: Lunch with Ed in the park. We've known each other for 15 years. He's the only person my age who is as devout as I am in my Catholic faith. I go to Mass two or three times a week, faith brings direction and purpose to my life.

1:15 pm: We're meeting up with friends, one of whom is younger, and married with two kids. I can't fathom that. I'm so focused on me, I'd leave my baby on the bus.

2:00 pm: Walking to football. I love summer, and the amount of fit girls in skirts and shifts is phenomenal. The standard of girls at football is definitely going up.

8:10 pm: At the pub with Ed's family. A traditionally good-looking girl joins us, and although I know she is pretty and quite nice, she does absolutely nothing for me. I tend to judge girls quite harshly that way – the 'If They Are Pretty, They Mustn't Have a Personality' logic, eh? All of my experience tells me this. Pretty girls use it to get what they want, so they don't need to have a personality.

9:35 pm: Thinking of Sam. It all went very quickly, jumping from stage to stage long before I was ready. I lost my virginity to her and now think it was a mistake. We have no contact. I am used to hoping that problems go away. I need to confront them if they're going to be sorted.

SUNDAY

10:00 am: Should really go to Mass but prefer to stay in bed for an indeterminable period, which seconds as a way of tricking myself into not doing any work, a real problem as of late.

12:04 pm: Joe, my little brother, phones. We chat about nothing really. I forget how right you are at 18, and how wrong everyone is.

3:17 pm: I'm retreating into myself as the day goes on. Now reading random rubbish and masturbating. I masturbate frequently, two times a day-ish. These are the points where I think that I am doomed to live this life forever.

5:00 pm: Been to Mass. Saw a really pretty girl there, and debated for the entire hour whether to speak to her. Decided no, as I thought God would be pissed enough that I wasted my hour imagining the girl. I really am the worst kind of Christian.

5:03 pm: Or maybe God would be happy she's Catholic. I'm inclined towards Catholic girls because it's a lot less explaining, and justifying why I do the things I do. My religion defines me more than anything. Not that I'm on a mission to convert the world to Catholicism. But it might help.

6:45 pm: Heading to Mum's. Girls have accused me of putting family before anything else, seeking their approval. This has been problematic, but validated by the fact that my family is still here. Girls are not.

8:38 pm: Spent an hour with Mum, probably the most important person in my world. I think that's still okay at 23. She's my little lighthouse in the dark, never presses for details. Just knows I need to be.

8:39 pm: Oedipus has got nothing on me.

10:39 pm: Finished the second draft of an email to Sam, my ex-girlfriend. Only last week did I realise what I did to her. Our relationship hadn't been working, but then someone close to me died, and I said I wanted time on my own, and she couldn't accept that, so I got nasty. When she wanted to talk about something one night, I said, 'Be quiet and go to sleep.' Not cool. In my letter, I wrote: *I was wrong to use that as a smoke screen; it was even worse to take it out on you.* That's pretty much what a bastard I am.

11:35 pm: Finished writing four quick poems, all about the same things: Sam, Suzy, my friend who died and Suzy.

1:19 am: Sunday insomnia. It only happens on Sunday when I know I need to be asleep for work. I trick my brain by thinking about girls I like and imagining a future. Today I make up a girl named Jessica. I will meet her on Friday when I go to a World Youth Day meeting, she is completely fictional, and you'll be pleased to know that she is completely happy.

1:35 am: Rereading poems from earlier.

MONDAY

6:00 am: First day back at work. I am not a morning person.

7:45 am: Fell asleep on train, as I often do. Awoke with a double morning-glory effect. Getting off the train was embarrassing for all concerned.

8:00 am: See Suzy. Decide that me and her being together is not a good idea. This thought was perhaps easier to swallow because we were walking in opposite directions.

10:10 am: Training with a woman who has come to talk to us about maths. She is not attractive, but I still imagine what she's like naked, and what she'd be like to be in a relationship with. Decide she's probably not the most exciting person in the world. Feel guilty for deciding in the first place.

1:00 pm: My kids are taking an exam. Thinking about how at work I am not a sexual being in the slightest. The women are all so motherly (apart from Suzy) that it just doesn't come up.

3:35 pm: Need to get out of the habit of looking at Suzy and thinking, 'You are amazing. Your smile, your eyes, your bum, your laugh…'

8:30 pm: Home and reading really crap romance novels. This is my ultimate guilty pleasure. I am outwardly very snobbish about books. (Favourite novel: *Wuthering Heights*.) But I like the fact that trashy novels all finish nicely and make me believe that that's a possibility.

9:30 pm: Home alone. In uni, I lived with two girls and another guy. It was one of those friendships where we were so close that it didn't matter what anyone else did or said; they were the centre. I miss that closeness.

10:00 pm: Suddenly very conscious that my life is essentially work + bolt-ons.

TUESDAY

8:00 am: Enduring teasing from Rose, a teacher who is like the coolest aunt you could ever have.

9:00 am: I was observed in class, and the observer says some really nice things about me. Awkward staff room situation, where I was just singled out for praise. Uncomfortable because others deserve the praise as much as me.

10:10 am: School assembly. Bored. Tallying which teachers look after me, and which let me try on my own. It's about 80/20. I need to grow up.

3:30 pm: Am stuck outside my classroom and waiting to get back in. Suzy is having a meeting with Claire, who is quite good-looking for her age. Her ex-husband was a prick. She doesn't deserve it, and hopefully she'll find someone. Maybe me, ha ha.

4:00 pm: In staff meeting. This is my favourite time of the week. I am pretty much allowed to be my favourite version of me – interrupting, impossible to control, sarcastic – and no one can touch me. I imagine this is how stand-up comedians feel, and it is an intoxicating rush.

4:15 pm: My colleagues pretend they don't like it, but generally I think I bring a smile to their face.

5:00 pm: Ella and Suzy and I just found out we are going ABROAD! We have a feeder school to visit. Free holiday! I love when it's just us three and we can laugh and just be. We're young, we're teachers, we have the same humour and politics. It's just bliss.

8:00 pm: Pub with Aaron, a schoolmate and very good laugh. He's always very honest. We speak about mutual friends, and then he tells me that I'm 'not horrible', but that my 'obnoxiousness comes out in random bursts', which can be 'disconcerting'. He also says that I'm so 'passionate' about everything I talk about that it can be 'weird'. His assessment is true. And not all bad, apart from the weird bit.

8:35 pm: I've just tried to set Aaron up with Suzy. I told him that if I don't get to be happy with her, then someone else should be happy with her – someone I trust. Aaron says that this is not a convincing sale.

—m—

EJECTED
FROM THE
RELATIONSHIP

9

BREAK-UPS & BEYOND

the divorcee rebounding after a 12-year marriage into the arms of a bloke who loves her a *wee* bit too much

36, FEMALE, LONDON

SUNDAY

6:30 am: Awoke early this morning next to a void, with that familiar ache: the disbelief that my husband of a decade is not here, that he's with someone else. I want it all back.

6:31 am: Yet I know it wasn't working.

10:00 am: My boyfriend has called twice, full of enthusiasm about us, as ever. We've been together a year, very on-and-off.

10:15 am: Just told my housemate that I'm not sure about the boyfriend. Her response: 'You could do a lot worse.' I know I could. It's wonderful to be loved. But I don't love him. I only seem to love the one I've lost.

12:29 pm: I really, really miss my husband today. I've missed him all day; it feels like a lung is gone or something. Reality: our arguments are over, our fingers are bare, our bed's empty, our stuff is in storage and our friendship is dangling by a thread. The latter seems to be reliant on the fact that neither of us has found anyone else who makes them laugh as much.

4:15 pm: I feel really shitty about all this uncertainty, this reboundery. One thing I should've learned by now is to just stop looking around and get on with it. Really, what can you do but enjoy what you have?

11:00 pm: My dreams don't help. The night before last I had a dream, and all I can remember is the bit where I sagely told someone: 'Don't sacrifice your marriage, not for anything.' I woke up next to the boyfriend and felt shitty.

11:10 pm: Text a response to Boyfriend. Texting means being able to talk less. It's lazy. I do it all the time.

MONDAY

6:50 am: Woke up thinking about Boyfriend and Husband, as usual. Husband's girlfriend is leaving this morning I imagine. I think that's their arrangement – just long weekends.

7:35 am: Boyfriend is coming to see me later on. I keep telling him we might not last, and that he must put all other considerations first.

10:00 am: Trying to work, but every single day I hope Husband is going to call and say he wants me back. It doesn't make any sense, but I miss him. I miss his arms, his chest, his nose, looking at him, hugging him. I really miss him physically. Which is amazing considering how much I pushed him away when we were together. I have to do loads today, so I hopefully won't think about it too much.

11:00 am: Boyfriend called to confirm tonight. I know I should just enjoy his company, and later on, the sex. With Boyfriend it's all so easy and nice. The only problem is I'm not ready for it. Like my housemate says, he's besotted. That's not easy to deal with when you can't reciprocate.

12:43 pm: Seem to be getting on well with people and work. I need to remember that it's going to take time to put down roots here. I've had a complete life change. Only 18 months ago I had my own home in the countryside, a husband and a decent job. Now I'm in a house-share in London, far from my friends. It's quite lonely, although usually I'm cool with my own company. I need to get out more, and be more busy.

1:00 pm: Interestingly, I am constantly thinking about Boyfriend anyway. We spend our time in a bubble – all romance and sex and lovely stuff, but we're always alone. I know it's not very *real*. And ultimately, not the relationship that will make either of us happy long term.

1:07 pm: Ahhh someone just sent me a cheesy email including, *Life is too short to wake up with regrets. So love the people who treat you right.* S'true, innit.

6:23 pm: Boyfriend is on his way over. I find he's very whiney lately. Naturally I blame myself. He's probably a bit needy in the face of my permafrosted heart.

9:00 pm: Instead of cooking a delightful meal, I felt the need to get hammered and drag him out for a dinner of peanuts and beer.

TUESDAY

8:03 am: Arrrrghhhhhh.

8:04 am: Boyfriend just left and I feel sick. Because of the peanuts–beer dinner, but also because I have been awash in a pool of gushy, soppy pillow talk for the last 12 hours, with only a brief pause for sex. Why does he have to keep hammering me with this?

8:15 am: He knows I hate it. It boils down to the fact that I never say, 'I love you' in case it will make him think I am more ready than I am. But I woke up feeling guilty, and have therefore suggested he come round again tonight. This is the never-ending cycle. I do like him, I just wish he'd change the record, but he's never going to, and neither can I.

8:25 am: I'm going to the park for a sarnie with my psychopathic one-time potential lover today. He's crazy but nice. Seeing a pattern.

10:15 am: My housemate just told me that I should play the field. For his amusement, that is. Having had a three-month dabble in the field last year – not long, as I can't stand being alone – I can testify that it's fun, but totally immoral. And I'm too old. Too old to be in this house-share + dating stuff. But then again, I was a bit young to be married + house.

10:16 am: My life has completely turned upside down. WTF.

11:34 am: Arse. My house purchase just fell through. So I am stuck in limbo. It took me ages to find the house so I'm gutted. Back to spending every spare hour with estate agents. Joy.

11:37 am: Upside: Boyfriend has just very sweetly booked us on a camping trip. I like.

4:55 pm: Sunny lunch with nice-but-slightly-crackers mate. Now I'd better do some work. Am determined to make up for last night's intolerance and general non-niceness by being super nice to Boyfriend this evening.

7:55 pm: Housemate assures me I haven't been horrible to Boyfriend. He says I've been provoked. I still feel bad. I think the prob is the fence-sitting, really. If I am not sure, I should face up to it ending. I just can't stand being on my own. Really finding it hard to adjust to not having an other half.

7:58 pm: I suppose it's all part of the grieving process. Very confusing. We were together for 12 years. We are best friends but not very good on the relationship level. Ding dong, Boyfriend's here.

WEDNESDAY

2:29 pm: Boyfriend just left. I was feeling reluctant to have any intimacy because my head was all over the place (guilt, guilt), but today I just realised the thing I love about this bubble of a relationship is that with him I can just switch off my thoughts and worries and let my body take over. Once his over-the-top mushy talking stops and I can relax my mind, it's just physical and that's something I've not experienced in a relationship up to now. Very simple, very animal and utterly blissful. Now back to work.

2:30 pm: I can't believe I spent the entire morning in bed.

6:32 pm: Just talked to my long-suffering friend. He asked how I am feeling about the men. I couldn't answer, so he did: 'Is it like you've been on a bender and woken up in a strange house, then realised there's no home any more?' That's exactly what it's like. He is wise.

6:34 pm: Email from husband. I am all hopeful. Every time. It's pathetic.

8:59 pm: Husband just rang up for a chat. That hasn't happened for a long time. I feel… challenged. I think that's the best way to describe it.

10:26 pm: It's really amazing how contact from him slings me up in the air and then slams me into the ground.

10:27 pm: Confidence: lost.

THURSDAY

8:14 am: Still feeling really low. However, I am a bit clearer. I can see why I feel the way I do about my marriage: I am suffering from grief, which is not the same as actually, rationally wanting the marriage back. I can see that without drastic changes in both of us, it's not going to work.

10:10 am: Thinking through last night's call. A couple of things he said remind me that he can be a bully. And childish. I didn't rise to the bait. I could see what the old pattern would have been: us against the world, him against me, me making his life misery. It's a load of crap. I've grown out of it. I just have to wait for the old emotions to catch up, I suppose.

2:00 pm: Nice emails today from Boyfriend, plotting fun things to do. And Husband has sent two emails today. Wonder what that's about. Maybe he's missing me too at the mo.

3:31 pm: Visiting another house. Like a huge disused shed on a plot of wasteland.

6:35 pm: Off to a party tonight. It's weird going out as a single. Nobody to hide behind! And the booze flows a bit too freely.

6:38 pm: All quiet on the relationship front. Unusual.

6:48 pm: Does everyone get this way before parties? The 'I don't wanna go' feeling? Honestly, I'd rather have my head flushed down the toilet at this moment.

7:35 pm: Boring me seems to be scoring a massive victory. Crap.

11:19 pm: I'm glad I didn't go. I'm pretty sure it would have got messy.

SATURDAY

10:56 am: Full of beans this morning. Went for a sunny early morning walk had a really good house viewing, had a go at some swings at the park and then good feedback at work.

12:15 pm: Had a nice chat with Boyfriend. He's ridiculous but sweet. He was supposed to be visiting friends up north with his kid this weekend, but has mysteriously decided that it's better to go to London. I know it's because he wants to see me. The only problem being that it is to the possible detriment of his other friendships.

3:00 pm: I really feel better about Husband since the phone call. Must see how that lasts. We might go out for an evening this weekend. Perhaps my stupid hope won't pop up: that he'll drop to his knees, declare great changes and undying love, and put my wedding ring back on. It took balls to get out of that marriage and admit defeat.

4:46 pm: Mmm, Boyfriend is coming to see me with his kid. This ramps the relationship up, and I wasn't expecting it. I feel very uneasy. Of course, when I visit there occasionally, fine. But I don't want to be included in the family picture unless I am sure about it. This is different.

4:54 pm: I'm going to go for a pint and a read of the paper. Nothing like it for blanking out the facts of life.

5:05 pm: My mother-in-law rang. She and I miss each other, so we are arranging to go out. Family invasion was a big issue in my marriage. When things went wrong, we seemed to disappoint them. Now I can't think of anything worse than taking a boyfriend 'home'. But I still like her.

5:30 pm: Boyfriend just called on speakerphone from the car, without consulting with me privately first. Glad I didn't lose my cool. I'm mellowing in my dotage, clearly.

9:30 pm: Went out with boyfriend and his daughter, and it was actually fine. He's quite considerate (read: keeps a lid on the gushing love talk) when she's around, and we all got on.

SUNDAY

12:23 pm: Received two lovely cards today, one from the boyfriend and one from my husband's sister. Feeling loved.

5:14 pm: Just went to a meet-the-author event. Lots of jaded singles there laughing at themselves. Quite interesting hearing the shite some people have gone through. Maybe I hooked a good one, judging by some of the stories. Or at least a guy who will see me through this part of life.

7:00 pm: Husband blew me out tonight. Quite glad. I'm still confused, but I think things are getting clearer. Chuntering on.

—ᴍ—

the geeky guy experiencing the post-break-up crazies

26, MALE, HAMPSHIRE

THURSDAY

10:26 am: It is a beautiful sunny day on the South Coast of England. The sun really improves my mood. Missing Amy, my girlfriend of six months, who I'll see next week. Looking forward to oral sex! I have only in the past year discovered how great it is to give oral sex! I'm not too fussed about receiving, but giving is a great pleasure to me and, hopefully, the other person.

10:28 pm: I have no job or commitments at the moment, which I think may be a problem in itself for me. Too much time to analyse my life and create problems that are not there. I need to stop worrying about silly little things. They may be silly, but they really do hurt me. Job interview on Monday.

1:33 pm: On Facebook. Facebook says I'm in a relationship with Amy. So that has to be true, right? I am in a relationship, I think. But she is scared, scared that I will leave her. I am scared that she is scared. I love being with her, we kiss, we cuddle, we make love – it is always so much more than sex.

8:28 pm: On MSN messenger with Amy. I find it much easier to talk to people over the Internet. She has a secret and won't tell me. I need to stop worrying about silly little things. They may be silly, but they really do hurt me.

8:32 pm: I don't know if it bothers me because I'm insecure, or just nosy. But it really bothers me. I am very insecure and worried that she doesn't love me.

9:54 pm: Never fight with your partner on MSN messenger. It makes things worse and things are taken so out of context.

9:58 pm: She's saying that we're both in negative spaces, her with the divorce over her head, and me with my constant battle against depression, and unemployment. And she thinks that we've spent the past six months only trying to make each other happy, and not focusing on life around us. She says we both need to sort out our own issues before taking on someone else's.

10:08 pm: I think I may be single in about five minutes.

11:04 pm: Yep. I am now single. ☹

3:19 am: Every second feels like an eternity. Why is it that when our hearts break, time stops moving?

5:02 am: Life just seems so dark and so pointless for these hours. I've been here before, and I know it will get better. But right now I am feeling so lost and disorientated that I just don't know where to turn.

FRIDAY

10:48 am: Another great sunny day here. Shouldn't it be dark for me? After breaking up with Amy? Six months feels like a long time with her, almost like a lifetime. But upon sleeping on it, looking past my denial I think that she makes sense. We're both fruit loops. We are both going through a lot of stress at the moment. We both need to sort our heads out.

12:55 pm: Everyone has a past, and ours, I guess, collided. I can become smothering. I know it's not nice to be smothered, but I tried so hard not to do it. And for her, she, I think, was just coming out of a divorce and scared of being hurt. It was easier for her to do it herself. This is a very hard situation to deal with, and I'm still trying to get my head around it at the moment.

4:30 pm: In the psychiatrist's office, looking at a magazine. I've never ever had a skinny, magazine-type girlfriend, and am not ashamed to say that. Society is a pit that creates its own rules. I feel my looks aren't all that great, I'm not too sure. But I think it has opened my eyes up to finding a girl that has heart. The relationships I've been in have brought me such happiness.

6:18 pm: So the psychiatrist went very well today! I am amazed, because past experience tells me otherwise (one told me I should just 'walk off' my depression). We talked for a great hour, and figured out that my life is basically wrapped in fear.

7:43 pm: Amazing what 24 hours can do. Just off the phone with Amy, and we both seem to be extremely upbeat about life. She will be moving home soon to start afresh; I've been considering a new university course. We spoke about us, and she said it is just something that will have to happen in time. I love that lady so much.

8:15 pm: Did I say that Amy may want to meet up Wednesday? I love her.

9:00 pm: Thinking about our first date. We met on a dating website, and things just clicked. Sex was so much more than sex, we laughed, we comforted each other well. But apparently somewhere in there she felt as if she was in a relationship for the wrong reasons.

SATURDAY

1:03 pm: Spoke to Amy earlier, and she said she loves me! Woo.

1:106 pm: I supposed love is a large word, which covers a lot of areas.

1:15 pm: I just know that when we see each other next, everything will be fine. Yes, we had an argument, but who doesn't? Things were said that needed to be said, and I think it can only help us.

5:10 pm: Amy is going out for a girly night with her friends.

9:19 pm: She hasn't gone out, she is staying in with 'great company'. Now I assume she means her cat, but my mind just keeps ticking over. What if there is another man there?

9:30 pm: She didn't confirm it was her cat when I mentioned it. I know she met a guy on the Internet at some point.

10:02 pm: People truly need their own space, and I should just accept that she won't always be there 24/7.

11:05 pm: I really don't understand my relationship. Maybe it is all in my head.

SUNDAY

8:56 am: So I figured out Amy's secret! She is going to be in a studio audience for a TV show. Why couldn't she just tell me? We had a massive argument over it and ended up breaking up, because I became persistent and wouldn't stop nagging. Bizarre.

8:58 am: I thought we had a respectful relationship that we were meant to be at least truthful and considerate to the other person.

9:13 am: Amy is sending me so many mixed messages. Telling me we can be friends, but that she loves me. I'm so confused.

12:00 pm: Sunday phone call with my mum. Oh, she's the motivation for the phrase 'three's a crowd'. In all my relationships, my mother has said things to make me doubt the strength of the relationship. One of my exes despises my mother, and gave her the nickname 'The Poison Dwarf'.

4:44 pm: Seems as if it really is over. My heart says so, so it must be. It's a damn shame.

5:00 pm: I'm telling myself that I get to focus on my own life now. Get myself sorted, be who I need to be, no chains. If I become more secure and dependent on myself, then surely I can have more positive relationships with the people who love me? And I can settle down and have the one thing I really want, a family,

5:35 pm: So I am going to quit smoking! It's been four hours already and I feel rather tense!

7:00 pm: I know I keep talking about Amy, but truly deep down in my heart, Maddy will always be the one. My first love. She was my rock. We were together for three years, and one day I ran away. I had a change of heart, came back, but had completely broken her heart. So I had to go back home to my parents'.

7:51 pm: Abstaining in masturbation is a rather extreme way to punish myself. I won't touch myself until things work with Amy again.

9:13 pm: Six months with Amy feels like a lifetime. And still I am wanting more.

10:15 am: As for abstaining from masturbation, I failed.

MONDAY

9:25 am: Amy messaged today saying that she enjoys my company, yet doesn't want to be friends. I'm very upset about this. I feel as if she is just running a hundred miles in the other direction to protect her own feelings.

9:27 am: Which is fair enough.

9:29 am: I may play her at her own game and make her realise what she is missing.

10:25 am: I guess today is the first day of the rest of my life! I need to focus and change. It's been almost 24 hours since my last smoke and am feeling good.

12:00 pm: Went for a three-mile walk this morning. Job interview today.

12:28 pm: I've started smoking again.

12:30 pm: What a fucking rollercoaster ride this week has been.

—⁂—

the new divorcee navigating girlfriend sex and ex-wife relations… while still living with his wife

66, MALE, GREATER LONDON

WEDNESDAY

4:50 pm: Rowing with wife about how I can afford to go away for the weekend. Of course she doesn't know that I'm spending it with GF, so I got on the defensive.

5:00 pm: Still rowing, just left in a huff.

5:10 pm: She just called, and I didn't pick up. Listening to the voice message, which is a complete harangue.

5:12 pm: She's calling again, which I'm ignoring.

5:25 pm: Email from the wife with info about a trusteeship she wants to apply for. She wants my help to compose an appropriate letter. There are so many inconsistencies in our relationship. We tried to get back together a few months ago, but it lasted three days before we were fighting again. I still love her, but our arguments always stem from money. It's always been a problem: she's from a wealthy background, and I have never made enough. Then I borrowed to try and satisfy her wants. Which of course made things worse.

5:30 pm: And then there's the GF. She has her own money problems stemming from business problems and an ex-husband, ex-boyfriend, mother, father, children and siblings who all create problems.

11:15 pm: Wife's lights are out, she is asleep. When I first found out that she had signed up to an Internet dating site, that seemed to give me carte blanche. She tells me that she finds it very difficult to find another man. I think she is beautiful.

11:17 pm: Fantasising erotically about women. One in particular, let's call her M. I met her on the same Internet dating site where I met GF, and had an intense couple of months. I was then unceremoniously dumped by an email, telling me that I 'wanted more than she could give and gave more than she could take.' Not happy, and ego-bruised. Still don't understand it.

11:25 pm: If I'm honest with myself, M was insatiable, but intellectually very boring.

THURSDAY

8:00 am: I'm writing this in the annex of the home I share with my wife of 40 years, from whom I've been technically separated for three. But under the same roof. The annex is not as luxurious as the house, but in the three months since I've moved down, our relationship is much better because we're no longer driving each other mad.

8:02 am: If we could get back together, I would be happier. A reconciliation would have to be on my terms: no arguments about money, and acceptance by my wife of me the way I am. I suppose that means I need to accept her the way she is.

8:05 am: I've been thinking recently that I need to think more deeply. Particularly about relationships. If I knew what I was looking for, I probably wouldn't be writing this.

10:30 am: At my business consultant job, an email from my wife about scheduling arrived. My wife is a pretty redhead. I still find her beautiful; I am ambivalent about her sexual allure, probably because of her dismissiveness towards me. She once told me that the curls I have at the back of my very thin head of hair are my only redeeming feature, though I think I look younger than my age. Not all the time.

10:59 am: An innuendo-laced text from my GF. She wants us to be rather closer mentally, as well as physically. She is in danger of getting a bit too clingy. She is my third, and the longest – ten months, aside from an interregnum when my wife and I tried to get back together a few months ago. Which was a disaster. While we like each other, GF does tend to want more of me emotionally than I want to give. I feel very uncomfortable, and occasionally guilty about it; do I call it off (again) or not? Every time I think I will call it off, I succumb to the 'pleasures of the flesh'.

11:00 am: Do I sound like a bit of a bastard?

5:00 pm: Thinking about sex. I am trying to understand why it is that my wife of 40 years and I couldn't really get it together sexually, even though we both claim to love each other. Meanwhile, my girlfriend and I have an amazing sexual relationship. I amazed both myself and my girlfriend when my first performance was, in her words, 'astounding', particularly considering my age and general lack of fitness. We have an amazing sexual relationship.

5:03 pm: For years, my wife complained about the lack of sex, and I was feeling so emasculated that I asked the doctor to prescribe Viagra. Which he did, and I never used.

8:08 pm: I'm chairing a public-speaking contest, and GF is in the audience. I feel remarkably remote from her. Nevertheless, I'm arranging for her to meet me in the West Country this weekend. I am spending Friday away on business, and we can therefore spend some time together over the weekend without actually 'going anywhere'. This is particularly relevant, as she's asked me to go with her to her house in Europe. It's in the wilds somewhere and I'm not keen.

1:15 am: I have to get up very early tomorrow for a crack-of-dawn meeting, but that isn't stopping me from going to bed late and fantasising erotically about having sex with any number of women I lust after. How can you tell your best mates that you lust after their wives/girlfriends? You'd not only lose your mates, but also the occasions to see the objects of desire, and, therefore, the ability to fantasise when you're not with them.

FRIDAY

7:15 am: Last night I fell asleep thinking about work today – didn't even think about GF. I told her last Saturday that I couldn't see her, but didn't say why. We did get together on Sunday for the staple diet of eating, drinking, Scrabble and sex, not necessarily in that order.

7:20 am: No messages or contact at all from GF. Usually there is lots of texting, particularly innuendo.

7:45 am: On the Tube. Worst day of my life was on the Tube a couple of years ago: I was standing, staring at a beautiful young woman. She was raven-haired and slim, with a wonderful figure and great legs. She saw me staring, smiled sweetly and asked if I'd like her seat.

3:00 pm: Spent the day away with colleagues, working out the company's value proposition. My team accused me of being tired and grumpy. Rather than explaining how I spent the evening, I explained that Pooh Bear said that being grumpy was what bears do.

6:33 pm: Sitting in a hotel in a small town in the west drinking Diet Coke, waiting to hear from GF what time she'll arrive before we drive down to the coast for the weekend.

6:43 pm: Business phone call interrupted me; knocked over Coke, fortunately over a lamp rather than my computer. Irritated barman is concerned he is going to get an electric shock cleaning up.

6:50 pm: GF just phoned; she's driving home from work, which means at least two hours before she gets here. GF has a very strange job schmoozing rich people and doesn't seem to get on too well with her colleagues, which makes her edgy at times.

7:04 pm: The bar/lounge is peopled by middle-aged men and women with middle-aged spreads. But I just noticed a girl/woman at the bar in what looks like a wedding dress. She has a very white back and reasonable figure, but is generally unappetising.

7:10 pm: A blonde woman asking for matches at the bar. Also unappetising. When I was in my early 20s, I went out with a similar-looking woman. She was a few years older, and she taught me a lot. I'm currently reading Stephen Vizinczey's *In Praise of Older Women*. Wouldn't be so keen now.

SATURDAY

12:15 pm: The touching, the stroking, the fondling, the exploration of orifices with every organ involved. Wow! My body is now reacting to these thoughts in what I suppose is a fairly predictable way. Great stuff.

8:51 pm: I am realising that I have wasted a large number of years out in the sexual wilderness during my marriage, satisfying myself purely by hand, turned on predominantly by viewing lesbian porn sites. It's amazing how a highly intelligent being like myself would turn to that stuff.

SUNDAY

11:00 am: A very hot couple of nights in the west. We did play Scrabble and each won two games. But we found time for some very energetic other activities.

1:15 pm: Daughter just called. The younger one is a terrific supporter of her old dad; the older one doesn't want to know, so I don't tell her where I am.

8:05 pm: Back home. I told GF when we got back that my wife and I are sort of talking about going away somewhere for Easter.

11:00 pm: How was the weekend? Absolutely amazing. Never have I enjoyed so much sex in so short a time. GF seemed to enjoy it too.

MONDAY

12:14 pm: Far too busy to think about sex today, although I did attend a board meeting for a company that specialises in alternative sexuality. Why I'm involved? I'm not sure. Probably the mental equivalent of extreme skiing.

5:08 pm: Getting really bored with the exchange of (angry) emails from my wife. They're really about nothing, but I can tell that there is huge anger in them. I don't know what I've done or not done, but to be honest, not much has changed after 40 years of marriage. It's never been a strong relationship. Our first argument was on our honeymoon night, and that was followed by years of my pursuing my career. It's always been very rocky.

5:11 pm: Anyway, I'm supposed to have our Easter trip all arranged, and I haven't. And now she's telling me that she's got a hospital appointment on Monday evening so we'd have to get back early, so it's no good going where we planned.

6:00 pm: Strange thing is, if my wife and I could get back together, I'd like to do so. But not with the relationship we've had for the last 20 years. It's all too ridiculous. Last time we tried reconciliation, it was a disaster.

—m—

the graduate student angry at her evil ex, while her best guy friend pursues her

25, FEMALE, NORTH YORKSHIRE

SUNDAY

8:00 am: Ha ha! Stuart wanted to take me home last night. I made it quite clear that I don't do one-night stands. I'm glad he wasn't offended. Though even if he was, I guess it doesn't matter. I have my pride and he's only a man.

9:00 am: I have been single since 12 weeks ago, when my boyfriend of seven months abruptly left me, saying he 'just needed to be single'. But six weeks ago he sent a text telling me that he was now in a relationship. My reaction wasn't very good, so he called. He admitted that he had been seeing her behind my back for well over a month. I was heartbroken all over again. Part of me still loves him and would give anything to have him back, but the rest of me despises his lying and putting my sexual health at risk.

12:11 pm: Well it turns out that The Slag is totally vile. She's ten years older than me. Part of me wonders why he would have left me for somebody so promiscuous and cold-hearted? But the rest of me feels glad that he's most likely going to get hurt.

3:15 pm: I shouldn't still be thinking about him. A man without ambition and without any prospects who lied. But I want him to feel like I felt. I loved him with all my heart and he lied to me for months.

7:27 pm: He's just sent me a text message, asking how I am. Every time I hear from him and every time I hear his name, my heart takes over and I want him back. I know that's stupid and I would never take him back, but I do miss him. Or at least I miss who I thought he was. It was an incredibly intense relationship. We were inseparable, rarely spent a night apart.

7:30 pm: Funny. I wonder why he is asking how I am? He obviously doesn't care. He proved that by sleeping with somebody else, and cheating and bullying me and ripping my heart out and stamping on it. God, don't ever let me fall in love again.

9:00 pm: Crying. I spend many nights this way, as I miss him. I need to think of the bad times. My friends tell me to meet men, and I do. They chat me up and proposition me, but what's the point, just so they can hurt me? I'm back up here on the shelf. The finest china is always left on the shelf and only brought down for special visitors. So, on the shelf I shall remain, until I find someone worthy.

MONDAY

8:30 am: Just woke wet with perspiration after a dream about him. I dreamt that I was going to a gig and they turned up. I hit her. Then he discovered what she was really like and begged me to take him back, to which I found great satisfaction in saying no.

8:32 am: The dream is probably a reflection that I'm going to a gig on Thursday, and I've been worried about bumping into them. I just pray that I don't see them as I know I'll either turn into a quivering wreck or Rocky.

12:54 pm: Checked my inbox on a dating site today. I get around seven messages a day. I check their profiles and only sometimes respond. Unless Jonathan Rhys Meyers begs for my hand in marriage, I imagine that I shall be alone for a while.

4:52 pm: Pub and chat with my good friend, Aidan. He's a wonderfully intelligent Oxford graduate. He knows *her* quite well, and says that when he meets her next week, he'll find out what the hell she thought she was playing at.

7:00 pm: Home. Just got a text from Aidan, suggesting we do something on Saturday. My ex always questioned Aidan's motives towards me, perhaps because he knew that he wasn't the only man ruled by his cock? He was bothered by our shared love of classic literature.

9:30 pm: Chat and a drink with my mother, who reminded me that he's a waste of space.

9:35 pm: I now realise that my mother had seen through him, and I should probably have listened to her. He hardly bothered with his family, only ever went to see his mother when he wanted something. At the time, I put my mother's disapproval down to the fact that she was afraid of losing me.

11:05 pm: I hate going to bed alone. I miss his arms around me and his face next to mine. I miss feeling safe and secure. I also miss the bloody sex. I think that maybe it is just loneliness, as I cannot possibly love him now that I've seen his true colours.

TUESDAY

11:44 am: Haven't really thought about him today. I think that I have only been feeling down because he contacted me. When there is no contact, it's easier. Difficult to go without it, though, when he was my best friend as well as my lover.

11:46 am: Last week, by the way, he sent me a text saying that he wouldn't be texting me anymore at was unfair to The Slag. Oh! But it was okay for him to *fuck* her while he was with *me*.

11:48 am: I really need to stop thinking about him, as I've loads of work to do and jobs to apply for.

5:49 pm: I have written a paper for university this afternoon, as well as part three of my short story, 'Hero Man and the Clay Penis', which I'm finding a great way to slag off the male species and vent my frustration.

6:01 pm: Looking forward to seeing that live band tomorrow. A combination of good music and a considerable amount of alcohol. I only want a decent conversation and possibly a dance. As soon as anything else is suggested, I'll make my excuses and leave.

6:04 pm: Was just thinking back to the last time I saw the ex. It was a couple of weeks after he had left me, and prior to his admission of infidelity. We went for drinks and then I stupidly agreed to go back to his flat. Obviously, we had sex. Five times, actually. Five times and I didn't climax even once. Although, to make things even, I ensured that he didn't either.

9:00 pm: Sat at home with my mother and the dog, who seem to have persistent coughs and matching flatulence problems. I'd give anything to be cuddled up on the sofa with my ex. Maybe a quick fumble during the ad break like we used to.

9:08 pm: Well, I've opened a bottle of Rioja. No doubt I'll finish it. The evenings are the loneliest. I know that I'm sat at home with just a bottle of wine to keep me company, and he's probably screwing the brains out of The Slag on my side of the bed. Bastard.

10:00 pm: The first thing I did when we split was order myself a new vibrator friend. For the first couple of weeks, Roger and I were inseparable. Now I have no desire to liaise with Roger Rabbit. Poor Roger may be feeling a tad neglected after a fortnight in my knicker drawer.

WEDNESDAY

11:45 am: Knobhead sent me a message this morning. He proposed on my 16th birthday. Diamond ring, a dozen red roses, the lot. Since then he has come crawling out of the woodwork every couple of years. Most recently, he was living with someone and had a child with her. Now he's come running back. Thing is, we've known each other 11 years. We can finish each other's sentences and I'm pretty sure we'd win 'Mr and Mrs.' But I'm not sexually attracted to him. I love him – like a brother.

12:43 pm: Friend on the phone, talking about anal sex. A no-no for me. I have no idea why a woman would agree; it is entirely for the man's pleasure, and I am *far* from giving a damn. Well, at least I know why he chose her over me. Ex said as much. I can add uphill gardening to her list of interests.

10:29 pm: He just sent me a text: *Spurs beat The Gunners. Good news x.* The Spurs are *my* team! He supports Man United.

10:31 pm: Another: *Just been on your blog and enjoyed. Brilliant.* I don't get it. Why?! *He* left *me*. Shouldn't he be busy shagging The Slag rather than texting his ex? Really annoyed.

10:33 pm: He told me about The Slag by text, by the way. It took him six weeks to admit he'd left me for someone else. I am still unsure as to how he found the time to form a relationship with her when we were rarely apart. I had keys to his place. Bloody men. Hang the lot of them.

3:30 am: I miss him terribly. Sat up crying.

THURSDAY

2:00 pm: Slept far too long. I cannot continue with this self-loathing. I need to believe that it wasn't my fault. I'm drinking too much and eating crap. He's already broken my heart and messed with my head, I can't let him affect my health. It's good I'm going out tonight.

8:15 pm: At a live band with my friends. They are fantastic.

9:37 pm: Just met a guy who my friend works with. I have never seen a more beautiful man. He's way out of my league, though. Men love the size-zero, fake-tanned, airhead type. I don't consider myself to be very attractive. Size 16 with DDs.

10:30 pm: Paul is here. I've known Paul for years. We're dancing.

12:10 am: I'm in Paul's room! We danced, had a kiss, walked to his – losing a pizza and a kebab in the process – had a fumble in his garden shed (random!), and then went to his room. So classy.

FRIDAY

10:30 am: Just got in. I broke my no-one-night-stand rule and succumbed to the evils of casual sex. Thoroughly enjoyed.

10:35 am: I never offered Paul my phone number. I simply searched for my clothes and asked him to show me out. I will not be ashamed. I've known Paul since I did my A-levels, so it's not as if he's some random stranger I dragged out of the pub.

3:15 pm: I will not be using a dating site again. Bombarded by messages. One particular gentleman asked if we could meet for a coffee. I said 'yes, just a coffee.' Five seconds later he's telling the world on Facebook that his life is finally 'looking up' and he may have found the one! No wonder he's on a dating site.

8:30 pm: Had a few beers with Aidan, who's been ever-so supportive of my split. My friends have been telling me for years that he's in love with me, but I never believed them. I think they may be right. I can trust him, and I'm starting to see him in a different light. Granted, I'm not physically attracted to him, but that is something which can change.

8:32 pm: He keeps dropping hints but never actually says how he feels. Maybe I should just ask him outright?

—◊—